MEDITERRANEAN DIET COOKBOOK 2021

DISCOVER QUICK & EASY, FLAVORFUL

MEDITERRANEAN RECIPES FOR

LIFELONG HEALTH

CATHERINE MOORE

DISCLAIMER

The information contained in the Book is for informational purposes only, and in no case may it constitute the formulation of a diagnosis or the prescription of treatment.
The information contained in the Book is not intended and should not in any way replace the direct doctor-patient relationship or the specialist visit.
It is recommended to always seek the advice of your doctor and/or specialists regarding any indication reported.

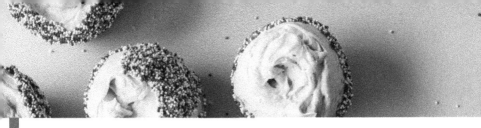

CONTENTS

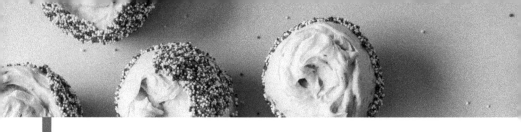

C O N T E N T S

INTRODUCTION

Mediterranean diet is basically the diet of nations living on the Mediterranean Sea. The diet aims to increase the intake of healthy fats, fruits, and vegetables and decrease the intake of saturated fats, red meat, sugar and sodium. It emphasizes an increased intake of whole grains, nuts, seeds, and legumes.

WHAT IS MEDITERRANEAN DIET?

●● — ● — ●●

First of all, it is important to know that classic Mediterranean diet isn't just food, but rather, it is way of life.

Mediterranean diet is based on simplicity and frugality. The main goal is to prepare food as close to natural state, as possible.

Mediterranean diet is more about lifestyle than diet. The main features are balanced nutrition, with lots of fresh fruits, vegetables, fish, olive oil, vegetable oils with low levels of animal fats, moderate consumption of wine (preferably red) with meals, and active lifestyle, in all aspects of life. Mediterranean diet is also known for its low glycemic index, low nutritional density, low consumption of saturated fat, and low consumption of cholesterol. It is also very high in antioxidant and low in omega-6 fatty acids cholesterol. Studies have shown Mediterranean diet is highly protective against cancer, cardiovascular disease and diabetes. It's also known for its beneficial effects on the microbiome. Mediterranean diet has been shown to improve certain aspects of health: physical, mental and emotional. There is strong evidence that Mediterranean diet affects hormones, inflammatory response, microbiome and endocrine system.

It can be harmful if is eaten in wrong quantities, consumed at inappropriate times or eaten for too many years

What to Eat?

Regarding dietary necessities, such as specific component, we can clarify that:

Mediterranean plant-based diet: adequate intake of plant foods, vegetables, fruit, cereal grain, legume and extra-virgin olive oil.

Mediterranean animal-based diet: adequate intake of species with the lightest fats (poultry especially the dark meat, and egg), grapes, grapes and other berries, seeds and nuts, wine, vegetables (especially the green leafy ones), some vegetables and fruits (like olives and varieties of grapes).

Mediterranean fish-based diet: sufficient intake of species with the lightest fats (fish, shellfish), pasta, olive oil and other foods to increase intake of fat-soluble vitamins K, A and D, vegetables and fruits.

Should we go on and mention that although Mediterranean diet is quite diverse, the diet is healthy, but not balanced. This of course, means that a lean person should not focus on the ratio of protein and carbohydrates (like a person with diabetes would usually do) but on the quality of what he or she is eating. Mediterranean Diet, in the future with more research and clinical studies) will be a paradigmatic example of healthy diet, with biological replicates which can be implemented in the western world. It's all about right balance with the right quantity of nutrients, the right quality, and the right time.

History of Mediterranean Diet

The Mediterranean diet is food patterns typical of the Mediterranean Basin, including southern Europe, northern Africa and Latin America. The origins of Mediterranean diet started with a study conducted by Ancel Keys in the 1970s, when he demonstrated that countries around the Mediterranean Sea had lower rates of cardiovascular disease than other parts of Europe. Thereafter, the Mediterranean diet was often connected with the lower rates of cardiovascular disease and cancer. Mediterranean diet is rich in fruits and vegetables, whole grains, legumes, nuts, and beans, as well as high in seafood, olive oil, and moderate in alcohol.

Benefits of the Mediterranean Diet

Here are the Benefits of the Mediterranean Diet:

This diet is known as perhaps the only one that provides you with good health in the long run. You will never feel hungry, nor will you feel as if though you are preventing yourself from eating delicious foods.

The only thing this diet requires is to reduce the consumption of unhealthy foods such as red meat, junk food, processed food, and sugars.

Mediterranean diet puts an accent on vegetables, fruits, seeds, fish, and legumes. You do not need to be a nutritionist or a doctor to know that a diet rich in such foods is a sure way to provide your body with healthy nutrients.

This diet is an extremely popular option for weight loss, but even if you are not willing to slim, you can switch to this diet because of the many health benefits it provides.

People who have heart and cardiovascular issues, skin problems, diabetes, or simply want to stay healthy and lower the risk of evil diseases (like cancer), are advised to start the Mediterranean diet.

Let's take a look at the health benefits that this diet brings.

Reduced Risk of Heart Failures
Providing your body with colorful meals that contain large amounts of fruits, vegetables, healthy oils, and lesser processed food or unhealthy ingredients is a sure way to remain in good health.

New England Journal of Medicine published a study in 2013 that was following more than 7000 people (men and women) in Spain who were suffering from type 2 diabetes. They were at high risk for cardiovascular illnesses; the ones that were following the Mediterranean diet (plenty of vegetables, fruits, fish, and olive oil) had about a 30% lower risk of heart failures. The researchers did not encourage the participants to exercise (the study wanted to see only the results of the diet).

The study reanalyzed the data in 2018, and they came with similar results.

Consuming large amounts of fish instead of red meat is the key to a healthy heart; the risk for seizures, heart attacks, cholesterol, and early death is reduced.

Prevents Alzheimer's Disease and Memory Decline

The Mediterranean way of eating will help your brain stay in good shape. As we get older, our memory tends to decline, and the brain's activity significantly drops.

The human brain needs food to function properly, and when that food is not suitable, the risk of diseases such as Alzheimer's grows higher.

Our brains need quality nutrients and oxygen, and the best way to provide that is by the right foods.

Food that is not providing our blood with enough oxygen will manifest in poor memory and cognitive functioning.

In 2016 the Journal Frontiers in Nutrition was monitoring the effect of the Mediterranean diet on the cognitive functions. The results showed that this diet does improve brain functioning and slows down memory declining.

Weight Loss and Healthy Weight Maintenance

Switching from a regular (mostly unhealthy) diet to the Mediterranean pattern of eating is a very common thing. This way of eating is not a new thing, nor was it created by nutritionists.

This is a regular lifestyle of the people who live around the Mediterranean (Spain, France, Italy, Balkan countries).

The menu consists of foods that are native to the area, especially fruits, vegetables, seeds, fish, nuts, herbs.

What makes this eating pattern so suitable for weight loss is the fact that it suggests consuming fresh and whole-food without additional additives that only add flavor and make you crave more unhealthy foods. The purging effect of fruits, vegetables, nuts, and healthy fats like olive oils cleanses your body from fat and cholesterol and helps in the slimming process.

The body is now provided with healthy nutrients that are easy for digestion. Healthy fats (olive oil, avocado, nuts) provide the brain and the body with sufficient amounts of energy, while the rest of the ingredients are not layered in fats all over the body.

Consuming this calorie-unrestricted Mediterranean eating pattern for five years will keep your weight balanced.

The food combination in its suggested amounts (daily, weekly and monthly) will result in a healthy weight loss.

If your goal is to lose a larger amount of weight, you can combine the Mediterranean diet with calorie restriction and physical activity.

Mediterranean Diet Helps in Managing Type 2 Diabetes

People who have type 2 diabetes are advised to follow diets that are not rich in carbohydrates and sugars. The Mediterranean diet might be a good solution for them, as well.

This diet is all about whole grains and healthy carbohydrates, which will not increase the blood sugar levels. Complex whole-grain carbohydrates (quinoa, wheat berries, or buckwheat) are a far better option than refined carbohydrates (white bread, sweets, juices, chocolate, fast food).

Studies show that people aged 50 to 80 years, who were diabetes-free and followed the Mediterranean diet for three to four years, did not develop the disease.

These people used olive oil and nuts, and in general, ate whole food and fish instead of processed food and meats. They had a 52% lower risk for type 2 diabetes.

Mediterranean Diet Reduces the Risk of Some Cancers

Food can be both cure and poison. When your daily menu contains foods rich in unhealthy fats (palm oil, butter), red meat, processed food, sugars, and large amounts of proteins (mostly from red meat) and carbohydrates (unhealthy options such as cookies, white bread, rice, French fries, etc.) – your body will suffer on the long run.

Most cancers are a result of poor eating habits, lack of physical activity, polluted air, and so on.

The Mediterranean diet helps in reducing the risk of cancers like colorectal, gastric, and breast cancer. The high intake of vegetables, fruits, and whole grains play a powerful role in keeping you healthy and in good shape.

Studies show that women who follow this diet (and use extra-virgin olive oil) have a 62% lower risk of breast cancer.

Mediterranean Diet Can Help with Anxiety and Depression

Almost everyone has experienced occasional depression (due to stress, problems in the family, or work).

Depression is a persistent loss of enthusiasm and enjoyment in doing things you once liked doing. Despair, lethargy, disinterest, sleeping problems are just a few of the symptoms of depression.

On the other hand, anxiety often manifests with nervousness before significant events, speaking to people, and meeting new people, going out, making mistakes, and fear of arguments. Sweaty palms, irritable bowel movement, overthinking, lack of sleep, and intrusive thoughts that you are not good enough or not doing things good enough are just a few of the symptoms.

Psychologists say that diet and mental health are tightly connected. Foods packed in healthy ingredients can seriously improve your general health, including your energy levels and mental state.

Suppose you avoid processed foods rich in unhealthy fats, red meat, white bread, and sugars. In that case, you will witness significant changes in every aspect of your life. Change of the lifestyle (new eating habits and physical activity) can improve the depression and anxiety symptoms. Good, healthy, and quality food impacts the mood and increases the levels of serotonin. When physical activity is added, depression becomes less severe. Naturally, you need to see professional help from a therapist, but your diet change could only bring positive shifts.

This diet also affects the immune system, which is one of the main factors in the risk of depression.

When your body is at a high risk of inflammation, it is more prone to depression. According to the studies published in The Journal of Clinical Psychiatry, depressed people have a 46% higher risk of inflammatory diseases in their blood.

The Mediterranean diet is packed with anti-inflammatory foods – olive oil, leafy greens, nuts, salmon, sardines, oranges, strawberries are just some of the foods that fight inflammation.

On the other hand, foods like margarine, red meat, processed meat, deep-fried foods, white bread, soft drinks (soda and tetra pack juices) are not recommended because they are not healthy, but because they are known for their inflammatory properties.

TIPS TO START OFF

The healthy Mediterranean way of life is all about eating balanced foods rich in vitamins, minerals, antioxidants, and healthy fatty acids. However, the Mediterranean diet is just one aspect of it. The Mediterranean way of life calls for regular physical exercise, plenty of rest, healthy social interaction, and fun. Balancing all these aspects was the secret of the good health of the Mediterranean folk back in the day. However, only the Mediterranean diet is the primary focus of this book. We will spend most of our time talking about just that.

Eat Healthy Fats

The Mediterranean diet is by no means a low-fat diet, but the fat included in this diet is considered healthy for the body, and the heart in particular. Remember: not all fats are created equal. Certain kinds of fats are healthy, while others do more harm than good. Monosaturated fats and polyunsaturated omega-3 fatty acids, for example, are considered healthy. Omega-6 polyunsaturated fatty acids and saturated fats are unhealthy.

These unhealthy fats are primarily present in most of the common food worldwide. The United States, for example, absolutely loves saturated fats. According to a survey, saturated fats constitute 11% of an average American's total calories, which is a very high number compared to an average Mediterranean resident, who consumes less than 8% of his/her calories through saturated fat.

If you wish to switch to the healthy Mediterranean way of life, the first thing to do is change the oils you consume.
Eliminating fats like butter and lard in favor of healthier oils like olive oil would be the place to start.

Consume Dairy in Moderation

We all love cheese. Dairy products are delicious, nutritious, and great sources of calcium. They should be consumed in moderation if you're following the Mediterranean diet.

It is usually a good idea to consume two to three servings of full-fat dairy products in a single day, where one serving can mean an 8-ounce glass of milk, or 8 ounces of yogurt, or an ounce of cheese.

Consume Tons of Plant-Based Foods

As we saw in the pyramid, fruits, vegetables, legumes, and whole grains form the basis of the Mediterranean diet. So, it is a good idea to eat five to ten servings of these in a single day, depending on your appetite. Eat as much of these as you want, but don't overeat. Plant-based foods are naturally low in calories and high in fiber and nutrients. Fresh unprocessed plants are best, so always be on the lookout for the best sources of these around you!

Spice Things Up with Fresh Herbs and Spices

Fresh herbs and spices make most of the recipes insanely delicious, while also providing health benefits. If you already use these in your daily cooking, more power to you! If not, we got you covered!

Consume Seafood Weekly

As we've talked before, one benefit of living close to the sea is easy to access to seafood. However, seafood holds a lower priority than plant-based foods in the Mediterranean diet and should be consumed in moderation. If you're a vegetarian, consider taking fish oil supplements to get those omega-3 fatty acids into your system.

Better yet, considering shunning your vegetarianism, and eating seafood to get the vital nourishment only seafood can provide.

Consume Meat Monthly

Red meat used to be a luxury for the Mediterranean people back in the day. Although not completely off-limits, you should try and reduce your red-meat intake as much as possible. If you love red meat, consider consuming it no more than two times per month. And even when you eat it, make sure the serving size of the meat in the dish is small (two to three-ounce serving). The main reason to limit meat intake is to limit the number of unhealthy fats going into your system.

As we talked before, saturated fats and omega-6 fatty acids are not good for health. Still, unfortunately, red meat contains significant quantities of these. As a beef lover myself, I eat a two-ounce serving of it per month, and when I do eat it, I make sure there are lots of vegetables on the side to satiate my hunger.

Drink Wine!

Love wine? Well, it is your lucky day. Having a glass of wine with dinner is a common practice in the Mediterranean regions.

Red wine is especially good for the heart and it is a good idea to consume a glass of red wine twice a week. Excess of everything is bad, and wine is no exception so keep it in check. Also, suppose you're already suffering from health conditions. In that case, it is a good idea to check with your doctor before introducing wine to your daily diet.

Work Your Body

Now you don't have to hit the gym like a maniac to work your body. Walking to your destination instead of driving, taking the stairs instead of the lift, or kneading your dough can all get the job done. So, be creative and work your body when you can. Better yet, play a sport or just hit the gym like a maniac. As I said at the start, you don't have to have to, but it will help... a lot.

Enjoy a Big Lunch

Lunch was usually the meal of the day when the Mediterranean residents sat with their families and took their time enjoying a big meal. This strengthens social bonds and relaxes the mind during the most stressful time of the day, when you're just halfway done with your work, probably.

Have Fun with Friends and Family

Just spending a few minutes per day doing something fun with your loved ones is great for de-stressing. Today, we don't understand the importance of this, and people feel lonely, and in some cases, even depressed.

Just doing this one thing has the power to solve a huge chunk of the problems our modern society faces.

Be Passionate

The Mediterranean people are passionate folk. Living on or close to sun-kissed coasts, their passion for life is naturally high. Being passionate about something in life can take you a long way towards health and wellness.

Planning Your Meals

Suppose you're a beginner and have not yet made the switch to the Mediterranean diet. In that case, you will need to identify what changes you need to make to your current diet to make it match closely with the Mediterranean diet.

In time, the Mediterranean diet will come to you naturally, but to start, you will need to plan. You will need to plan your portion sizes, and how often you eat certain foods. The changes are small but will benefit you in the long run.

Importance of Meal Planning

Meal planning is all about creating a road map for what you're going to eat, when you will prepare the food, and what ingredients you will need to buy. It might sound simple, but will save you from many headaches and make your transition to the Mediterranean diet much smoother. Meal planning is vital because:

- It enables you to be efficient with your time
- It enables you to plan what ingredients you will buy and when so that when you cook them, they are at their freshest
- You don't have to worry about what to cook multiple times per day. You take care of it in one sitting.
- It saves money by reducing food wastage. You cook everything you buy while it is still fresh.

Meal Planning Techniques

Meal planning is a flexible process, and every person has a unique way of going for it. You will eventually discover how you like to plan your meals, but it would be useful to look at a few templates of the common ways of doing it.

If you like to be moderately thorough and detailed, you can sit down and write what you will eat for breakfast, lunch, and dinner for each day of the week. If you like to munch on snacks from time to time, make sure you write those down too. Make sure the recipes you choose for that week are in season, and you can procure fresh ingredients for the written recipes.

• Suppose you like to get all the thinking for the whole month done in a single sitting. In that case, you can prepare meal plans for multiple weeks, along with shopping lists that specify what you will buy, and when, in such a way that the ingredients are at their freshest at the time of cooking. This will take a while, but a good place to start if you have the time. Just make sure you don't plan for too long, and make a new plan with every season to get the good seasonal stuff.

• Once you get slightly well acquainted with the diet, you will start to have the Mediterranean staples in your pantry at all times, and you don't need to plan all three meals per day or even your shopping list. You will have your favorite recipes that you will automatically shuffle as per your convenience. You will start to make larger batches so you can eat leftovers later if you're not in the mood to cook again. You might need to plan your big dinners once in a while, but that is about it.

In a nutshell, Mediterranean cooking will come to you naturally and will require minimal planning. Another great idea to keep in mind when you are on such a diet is to make a great shopping list. It will help you buy the right ingredients. Choose organic products if you can but only if they suit your budget. Your shopping list must include:

• Veggies like kale, garlic, spinach, arugula, onions, carrots

• Fruits like grapes, oranges, apples and bananas

• Berries like blueberries, strawberries, raspberries

• Frozen veggies

• Grains like whole-grain pasta, whole-grain breads

• Legumes like beans, lentils, chickpeas

• Nuts like walnuts, cashews, almonds

• Seeds like pumpkin seeds and sunflower seeds

• Condiments like turmeric, cinnamon, salt, pepper

- Shrimp and shellfish

- Fish like mackerel, trout, tuna, salmon and sardines

- Cheese
- Yogurt and Greek yogurt
- Potatoes and sweet potatoes
- Chicken

- Eggs
- Olives
- Olive oil and avocado oil

If you buy healthy and adequate ingredients, you will most certainly eat the right foods and you will definitely stay on your diet.

THE MEDITERRANEAN DIET PYRAMID AND SHOPPING LIST

Mediterranean Diet Pyramid

The Mediterranean Diet Pyramid is a nutritional guide that was developed by the World Health Organization in 1993. It was also worked on by the Harvard School of Public Health, and the Oldways Preservation Trust. It is a visual tool that summarizes the Mediterranean Diet's suggested eating pattern and gives a guide to how frequently specific tools should be eaten. This allows you to break healthy eating habits and not overfill yourself with too many calories.

How is the pyramid laid out? Let's go over each tier.

Olive oil, fruits, vegetables, whole grains, legumes, beans, nuts & seeds, spices & herbs:

These are the types of food that form the Mediterranean pyramid base. You'll notice that these are mostly from plant sources. You should try and include a few variations of these items into each meal you eat. Olive oil should be the main fat you use in your cooking and your dishes, so replace any other butter or cooking oil you used to use. Generous uses of herbs and spices are also encouraged to season your food and add flavor as an alternative to salt. If you don't have access to fresh herbs, you can buy the dried version.

Always be sure to read the nutrition labels to ensure no other ingredients are mixed with the herbs. Fresh ginger and garlic are also great flavor enhancers for your meals. They can be easily stored in the freezer.

Fish & seafood: These are important staples of the Mediterranean diet that should be consumed often as a protein source. You want to try and include these in your diet at least two times a week.

Try new varieties of fish, either frozen or fresh. Also incorporate seafood like mussels, crab, and shrimp into your diet. Canned tuna is also great to include on sandwiches or toss in a salad with fresh vegetables.

Cheese, yogurt, eggs & poultry: These ingredients should be consumed in more moderate amounts when on the Mediterranean diet. Depending on the food, they should be used sparingly throughout the week. Remember that if you are using eggs in baking or cooking, those will also be counted in your weekly limit. You want to stick to more healthy cheese like Parmesan, ricotta, or feta that you can add as a topping or garnish on your dishes.

Red meat & sweets: These items will be consumed less frequently when on the Mediterranean diet. If you are eating them, you want to be sure it is only in small quantities and prefer lean meat versions with less fat. Most studies recommend a maximum of 12 to 16 ounces per month.

You can still have red meat on occasion to add some variety to your diet, but you want to reduce how often you have it. That's because of all the health concerns that come with sugar and red meat. The Mediterranean diet is working to improve cardiovascular health and reduce blood pressure, while red meat tends to be dangerous in cardiac health. Greece's residents ate very little red meat and instead had fish or seafood as their main source of protein.

Water: The Mediterranean diet encourages you to be hydrated, which means drinking more than your daily intake of water. The Institute of Medicine recommends a total of 9 cups each day for women, and 13 cups for men. If a woman is pregnant or breastfeeding, that number should be increased.

Wine: Moderate consumption of wine with meals is encouraged on the Mediterranean diet. Studies have shown that moderate consumption of alcohol can reduce the risk of heart disease. That can mean about 1 glass per day for women. Men tend to have higher body mass so they can consume 1 to 2 glasses. Please keep in mind what your doctor would recommend regarding wine consumption based on your health and family history.

Your Mediterranean Diet Shopping List

Includes:

Extra virgin and virgin olive oils: These will be the least processed and refined versions of olive oil on the market. They will contain the highest level of plant compounds called "phenols" that act as antioxidants in the body. It might be a little pricier than the oil you used before, but it's well worth it when you're aware of the health benefits you will gain! This will be your go-to when it comes to cooking, frying, seasoning, and as the base of your salad dressings. Remember, less is more!

Vegetables: You have pretty much free rein with vegetables though if you can stick to low-calorie ones, that's even better for your weight loss goals. Vegetables like zucchini, mushrooms, cabbage, cauliflower, bell pepper, and spinach are low in calories. However, they are still very filling and high in fiber. Try new vegetables and eat them in different ways like a green smoothie or different salad combinations to get bored. Try to buy in season items so you can save yourself some money!

Fruits: Fruits are encouraged and are great as a substitute healthy dessert to treat yourself to. Figs and pomegranates are native to the Mediterranean area, but any fruit will do! Be sure to include various colorful fruits and vegetables which allow you to have a diverse range of essential vitamins and minerals. If you have diabetes, try and consume fruits that are low on the glycemic index such as oranges, apples, grapefruits, pears, or plums.

Legumes & beans: These are a great hidden source of protein which often get overlooked in the West in favor of red meat or poultry items. Thankfully, the Mediterranean diet urges you to try different variations of protein sources! Whether it's black beans, kidney beans, chickpeas, or lentils, these are great to experiment with. Don't forget hummus! These are packed with fiber as well, so they allow you to feel full for longer. Be sure you drink plenty of water to avoid constipation!

Whole grain breads and cereal: Whether it's rice, barley, oats, leek rice, quinoa, whole grain pasta, or whole grain bread, you want to be sure you are focused on whole grains that are healthier rather than refined or processed grains. Same goes with cereal. Be sure you read the label and ensure the product is made from whole grain starches and are not processed into refined products. Ezekiel bread is a whole grain bread made with no sugar. One slice is packed with fiber and contains only 80 calories! The trick with whole grains is that you can eat a smaller portion than you would with refined wheat products but stay full longer. These are also low on the glycemic index scale which makes them safe for diabetes patients.

Nuts & seeds: This includes cashews, pistachios, walnuts, sunflower seeds, pine nuts, flax seeds, almonds, and other nuts which may be your favorites. Keep these as a healthy snack throughout the day but be sure to avoid the chocolate-covered or salted versions which are unhealthy. You want to stick to the raw nuts. Chia seeds are also tiny but powerful! In just 2 tablespoons, you can have 11 grams of fiber! These are great to add to a smoothie or topping on oatmeal or cereal to fill you up. The great thing is they're almost flavorless so anyone can incorporate them into their meals!

Low-fat dairy: If you are used to dairy products in your diet, you don't have to cut them out entirely but you should switch to low-fat versions. Use fat-free yogurt or low-fat cheese, and switch to skim or reduced fat milk. On the Mediterranean diet you want most of your dairy calories to come from healthy cheeses like feta, brie, Greek yogurt, or Parmesan.

Herbs & spices: These are great to season your food with and add a great distinct flavor other than salt. You can try using fresh herbs like rosemary and parsley though they may not last as long in your refrigerator. You can always start a windowsill herb garden which are easy to maintain! If not, don't be intimidated and feel free to use dried herbs from the spice aisle. Experiment with new flavors that will enhance your flavor profile. Fresh garlic and ginger are also great flavor enhancers and considered essentials of Greek and Mediterranean cuisine. They have multiple health benefits and pack your meals with flavor.

Excludes:

Red meat: As we mentioned, you want to go light on red meat portions when shopping for your Mediterranean diet. If you want to get a few pieces, be sure they're smaller sized and lean meat cuts with less fat. Try only to have it once a week and keep an eye on your portion size. Also, avoid high-fat processed meats like pre-made sausages or hot dogs loaded with preservatives and high in sodium. These tend to cause inflammation in the body.

Poultry:

Again, you want to use poultry in your diet less often than you would on other diets. More lean cuts with less fat can be used now and then as long as you have smaller portions. For the most part, try and substitute your red meat and poultry meals with fish or seafood, although it's okay to have them once in a while during the week. Turkey or duck would be a healthier alternative to chicken because they contain less fat.

Refined grains:

These include things like bagels, cereal, or white bread that we might previously consider staples in our diet. But these should be excluded from your shopping list unless you have verified that the cereals, pasta, or bread are whole grain certified products.

Sugars: That means skipping things like candy, chocolate, ice cream, sugary juices, and sodas! Instead, try and treat yourself to berries or fruit as a sweet treat, or enhance your water with lemon or mint leaves for more flavor. Get used to the habit of having natural sugars in fruit as a dessert instead of wanting unhealthy baked goods.

Trans or saturated fats: Exclude things like butter or margarine which contain unhealthy saturated fats. You want to substitute any unhealthy oils like canola oil or vegetable oil with the healthier option of extra virgin olive oil. You want to use this in your cooking, frying, and as your vinaigrettes' main component.

Highly processed foods: These should be avoided on the Mediterranean diet. The rule of thumb should be if it comes in a box, you can't have it! That's because food that tends to be marked as "low-fat" or "diet friendly" is very processed and unhealthy for you. Instead of eating those empty calories, focus on what you can eat as a filling snack like some of the items we mentioned above.

Yogurt Peppers Mix

Prep Time: 10 min   **Cooking Time:** 15 min   **Servings:** 4

Ingredients:

- red bell peppers, cut into thick strips 2 tablespoons olive oil
- shallots, chopped
- 3 garlic cloves, minced
- Salt and black pepper to the taste
- ½ cup Greek yogurt
- 1 tablespoon cilantro, chopped

Directions:

1. Heat up a pan with the oil over medium heat, add the shallots and garlic, stir and cook for 5 minutes.
2. Add the rest of the ingredients, toss, cook for 10 minutes more, divide the mix between plates and serve as a side dish.

Nutrition:

calories 274, fat 11, fiber 3.5, protein 13.3, carbs 6.5

Cucumber Bites

Prep Time: 10 min   **Cooking Time:** 0 min   **Servings:** 12

Ingredients:

- 1 English cucumber, sliced into 32 rounds 10 ounces hummus
- 16 cherry tomatoes, halved
- 1 tablespoon parsley, chopped 1 ounce feta cheese, crumbled

Directions:

1. Spread the hummus on each cucumber round, divide the tomato halves on each, sprinkle the cheese and parsley on to and serve as an appetizer.

Nutrition:

calories 162, fat 3.4, fiber 2, carbs 6.4, protein 2.4

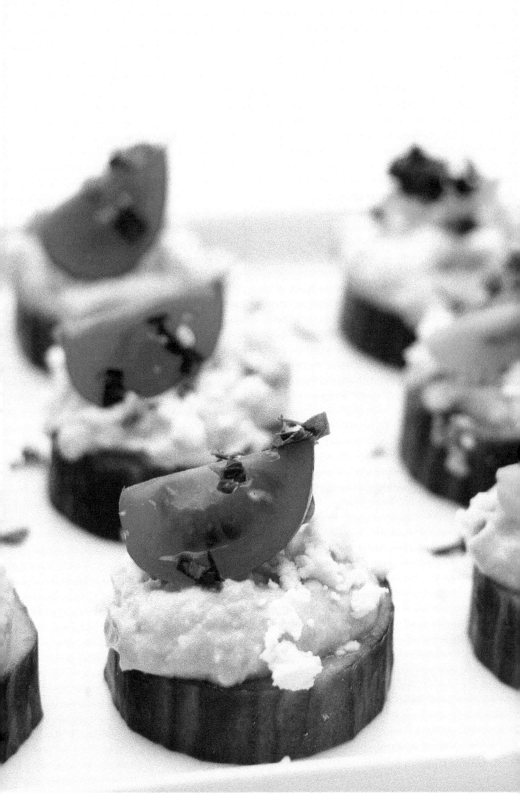

Cauliflower Quinoa

Prep Time: 5 min   **Cooking Time:** 10 min   **Servings:** 4

Ingredients:

- 1 and ½ cups quinoa, coked 3 tablespoons olive oil
- 3 cups cauliflower florets 2 spring onions, chopped
- Salt and pepper to the taste
- 1 tablespoon red wine vinegar 1 tablespoon parsley, chopped 1 tablespoon chives, chopped

Directions:

1. Heat up a pan with the oil over medium-high heat, add the spring onions and cook for 2 minutes.

2. Add the cauliflower, quinoa and the rest of the ingredients, toss, cook over medium heat for 8-9 minutes, divide between plates and serve as a side dish.

Nutrition:

calories 220, fat 16.7, fiber 5.6, carbs 6.8, protein 5.4

Baby Squash and Lentils Mix

Prep Time: 10 min   **Cooking Time:** 10 min   **Servings:** 4

Ingredients:

- tablespoons olive oil
- ½ teaspoon sweet paprika
- 10 ounces baby squash, sliced 1 tablespoon balsamic vinegar
- 15 ounces canned lentils, drained and rinsed Salt and black pepper to the taste
- 1 tablespoon dill, chopped

Directions:

1. Heat up a pan with the oil over medium heat, add the squash, lentils and the rest of the ingredients, toss and cook over medium heat for 10 minutes.

2. Divide the mix between plates and serve as a side dish.

Nutrition:

calories 438, fat 8.4, fiber 32.4, carbs 65.5, protein 22.4

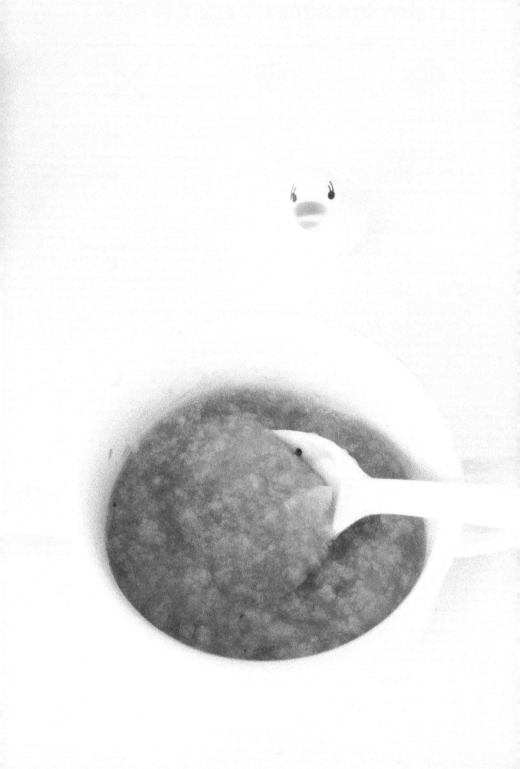

Basil Artichokes

Prep Time: 10 min   **Cooking Time:** 12 min   **Servings:** 4

Ingredients:

- red onion, chopped
- garlic cloves, minced
- Salt and black pepper to the taste
- ½ cup veggie stock
- 10 ounces canned artichoke hearts, drained 1 tablespoon olive oil
- teaspoon lemon juice
- tablespoons basil, chopped

Directions:

1. Heat up a pan with the oil over medium high heat, add the onion and the garlic, stir and sauté for 2 minutes.

2. Add the artichokes and the rest of the ingredients, toss, cook for 10 minutes more, divide between plates and serve as a side dish.

Nutrition:

calories 105, fat 7.6, fiber 3, carbs 6.7, protein 2.5

Rosemary Red Quinoa

Prep Time: 10 min **Cooking Time:** 25 min **Servings:** 6

Ingredients:

- 4 cups chicken stock
- 2 cups red quinoa, rinsed 1 red onion, chopped
- 2 tablespoons olive oil
- 1 tablespoon garlic, minced
- 1 teaspoon lemon zest, grated 2 tablespoons lemon juice
- Salt and black pepper to the taste 2 tablespoons rosemary, chopped

Directions:

1. Heat up a pan with the oil over medium heat, add the onion and the garlic and sauté for 5 minutes.

2. Add the quinoa, the stock and the rest of the ingredients, bring to a simmer and cook for 20 minutes stirring from time to time.

3. Divide the mix between plates and serve.

Nutrition:

calories 193, fat 7.9, fiber 1.4, carbs 5.4, protein 1.3

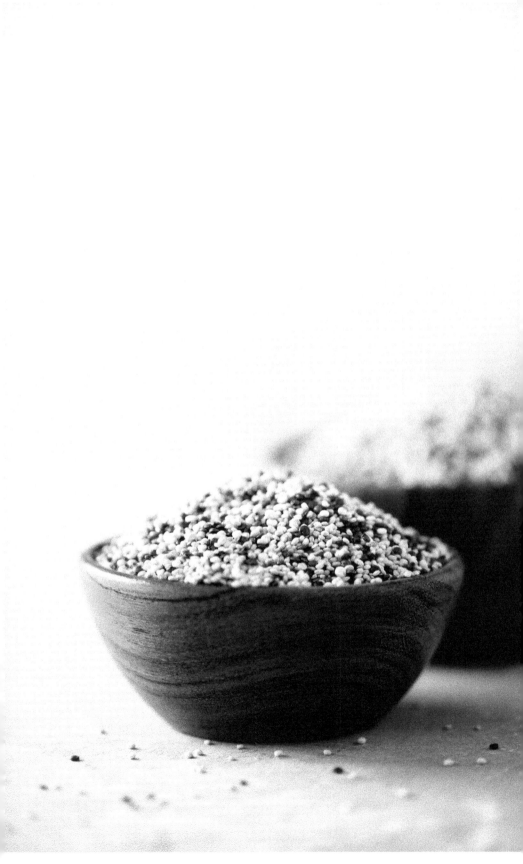

White Bean Dip

Prep Time: 10 min   **Cooking Time:** 0 min   **Servings:** 4

Ingredients:

- 15 ounces canned white beans, drained and rinsed
- 6 ounces canned artichoke hearts, drained and quartered 4 garlic cloves, minced
- 1 tablespoon basil, chopped 2 tablespoons olive oil
- Juice of ½ lemon
- Zest of ½ lemon, grated
- Salt and black pepper to the taste

Directions:

1. In your food processor, combine the beans with the artichokes and the rest of the ingredients except the oil and pulse well.
2. Add the oil gradually, pulse the mix again, divide into cups and serve as a party dip.

Nutrition:

calories 274, fat 11.7, fiber 6.5, carbs 18.5, protein 16.5

Parmesan Quinoa and Mushrooms

Prep Time: 10 min   **Cooking Time:** 20 min   **Servings:** 4

Ingredients:

- cup quinoa, cooked
- ½ cup chicken stock
- tablespoons olive oil
- 6 ounces white mushrooms, sliced
- teaspoon garlic, minced
- Salt and black pepper to the taste
- ½ cup parmesan, grated
- tablespoons cilantro, chopped

Directions:

1. Heat up a pan with the oil over medium heat, add the garlic and mushrooms, stir and sauté for 10 minutes.

2. Add the quinoa and the rest of the ingredients, toss, cook over medium heat for 10 minutes more, divide between plates and serve as a side dish.

Nutrition:
calories 233, fat 9.5, fiber 6.4, carbs 27.4, protein 12.5

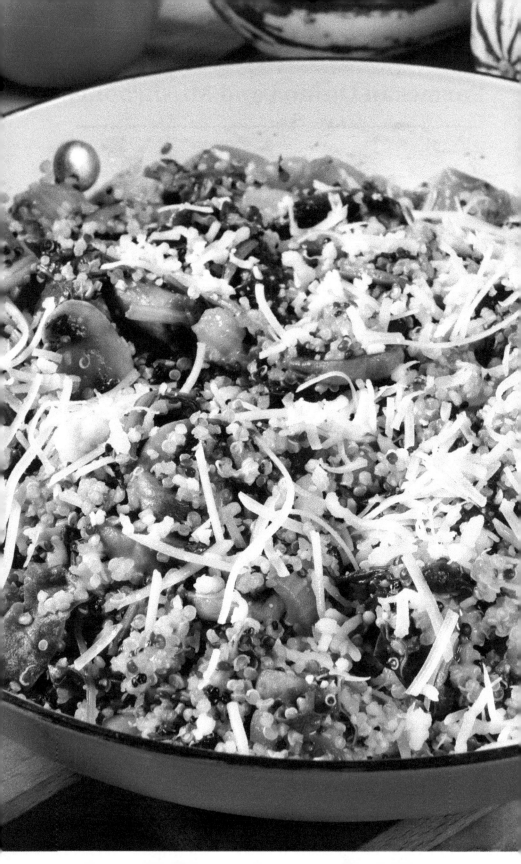

Herbed Cucumber and Avocado Mix

Prep Time: 10 min   **Cooking Time:** 0 min   **Servings:** 4

Ingredients:

- cucumbers, sliced
- avocados, pitted, peeled and cubed 1 tablespoon lemon juice
- tablespoons olive oil
- 2 teaspoons balsamic vinegar 1 teaspoon dill, dried
- 1 tablespoon cilantro, chopped 1 tablespoon chives, chopped 1 tablespoon basil, chopped
- 1 tablespoon oregano, chopped

Directions:

1. In a bowl, mix the cucumbers with the avocados with the rest of the ingredients, toss and serve as a side dish.

Nutrition:

calories 343, fat 9.6, fiber 2.5, carbs 16.5, protein 7.4

Lemon Endives

Prep Time: 10 min   **Cooking Time:** 35 min   **Servings:** 4

Ingredients:

- Juice of 1 and ½ lemons
- Salt and black pepper to the taste 3 tablespoons olive oil
- ¼ cup veggie stock
- 4 endives, halved lengthwise 1 tablespoon dill, chopped

Directions:

1. In a roasting pan, combine the endives with the rest of the ingredients, introduce in the oven and cook at 375 degrees F for 35 minutes.

2. Divide the endives between plates and serve as a side dish.

Nutrition:

calories 221, fat 5.4, fiber 6.4, carbs 15.4, protein 14.3

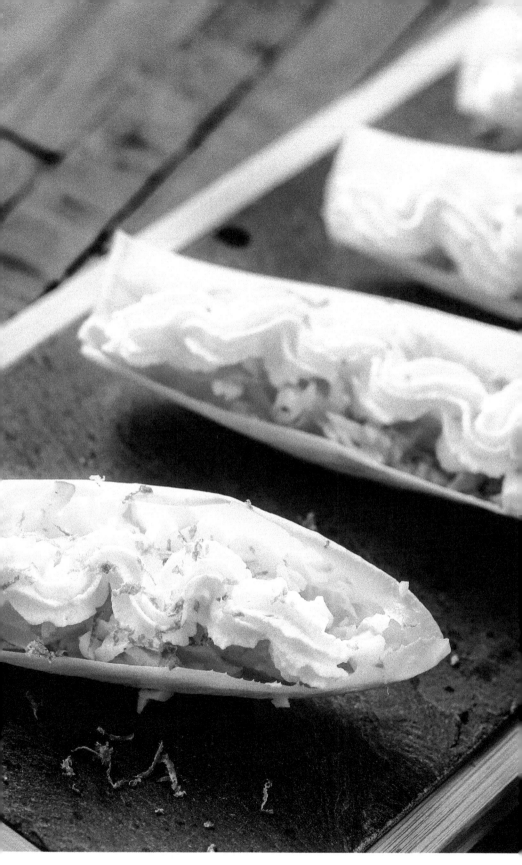

Garlic Snap Peas Mix

Prep Time: 10 min   **Cooking Tim:** 10 min   **Servings:** 4

Ingredients:

- ½ cup walnuts, chopped 2 teaspoons lime juice
- ¼ cup olive oil
- 1 and ½ teaspoons garlic, minced
- ½ cup veggie stock
- pound sugar snap peas
- Salt and black pepper to the taste 1 tablespoon chives, chopped

Directions:

1. Heat up a pan with the stock over medium heat, add the snap peas and cook for 5 minutes.

2. Add the rest of the ingredients except the chives, cook for 5 minutes more and divide between plates.

3. Sprinkle the chives on top and serve as a side dish.

Nutrition:

calories 200, fat 7.6, fiber 3.5, carbs 8.5, protein 4.3

Oregano Potatoes

Prep Time: 10 min   **Cooking Time:** 40 min   **Servings:** 4

Ingredients:

- 6 red potatoes, peeled and cut into wedges Salt and black pepper to the taste
- 2 tablespoons olive oil
- 1 teaspoon lemon zest, grated 1 teaspoon oregano, dried
- tablespoon chives, chopped
- ½ cup chicken stock

Directions:

1. In a roasting pan, combine the potatoes with salt, pepper, the oil and the rest of the ingredients except the chives, toss, introduce in the oven and cook at 425 degrees F for 40 minutes.

2. Divide the mix between plates, sprinkle the chives on top and serve as a side dish.

Nutrition:

calories 245, fat 4.5, fiber 2.8, carbs 7.1, protein 6.4

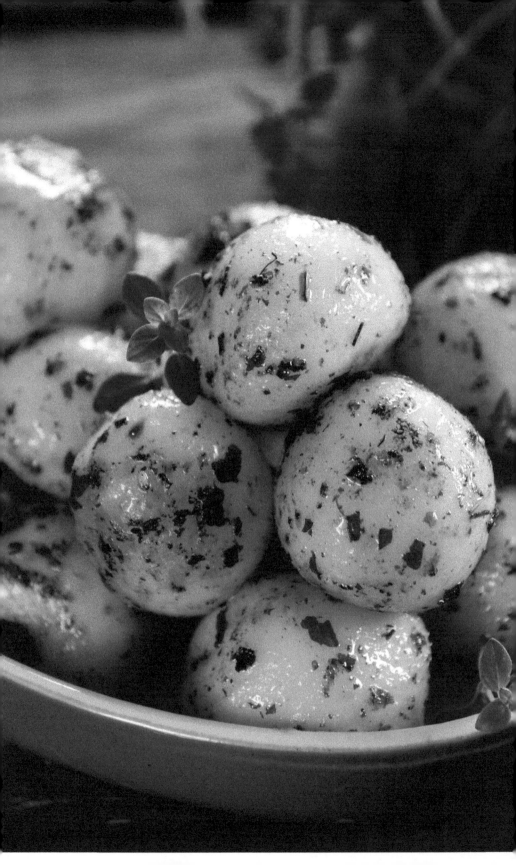

Chives Rice Mix

Prep Time: 5 min   **Cooking Time:** 5 min   **Servings:** 4

Ingredients:

- tablespoons avocado oil 1 cup Arborio rice, cooked
- 2 tablespoons chives, chopped Salt and black pepper to the taste 2 teaspoons lemon juice

Directions:

1. Heat up a pan with the avocado oil over medium high heat, add the rice and the rest of the ingredients, toss, cook for 5 minutes, divide the mix between plates and serve as a side dish.

Nutrition:

calories 236, fat 9, fiber 12.4, carbs 17.5, protein 4.5

Eggplant Dip

Prep Time: 10 min   **Cooking Time:** 40 min   **Servings:** 4

Ingredients:

- eggplant, poked with a fork 2 tablespoons tahini paste
- tablespoons lemon juice 2 garlic cloves, minced
- tablespoon olive oil
- Salt and black pepper to the taste 1 tablespoon parsley, chopped

Directions:

1. Put the eggplant in a roasting pan, bake at 400 degrees F for 40 minutes, cool down, peel and transfer to your food processor.

2. Add the rest of the ingredients except the parsley, pulse well, divide into small bowls and serve as an appetizer with the parsley sprinkled on top.

Nutrition:

calories 121, fat 4.3, fiber 1, carbs 1.4, protein 4.3

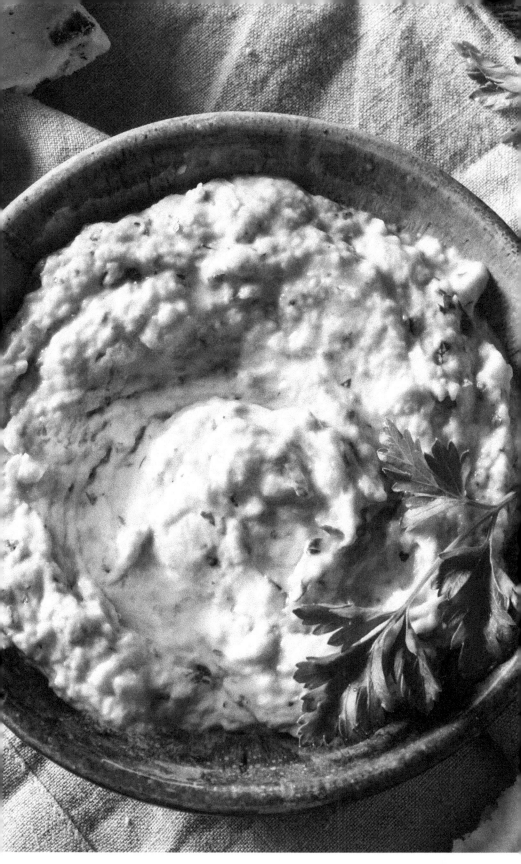

Hummus with Ground Lamb

Prep Time: 10 min   **Cooking Time:** 15 min   **Servings:** 8

Ingredients:

- 10 ounces hummus
- 12 ounces lamb meat, ground
- ½ cup pomegranate seeds
- ¼ cup parsley, chopped 1 tablespoon olive oil Pita chips for serving

Directions:

1. Heat up a pan with the oil over medium-high heat, add the meat, and brown for 15 minutes stirring often.

2. Spread the hummus on a platter, spread the ground lamb all over, also spread the pomegranate seeds and the parsley and sere with pita chips as a snack.

Nutrition:

calories 133, fat 9.7, fiber 1.7, carbs 6.4, protein 5.4

Red Pepper Tapenade

Prep Time: 10 min   **Cooking Time:** 0 min   **Servings:** 4

Ingredients:

- 7 ounces roasted red peppers, chopped
- ½ cup parmesan, grated 1/3 cup parsley, chopped
- 14 ounces canned artichokes, drained and chopped 3 tablespoons olive oil
- ¼ cup capers, drained
- 1 and ½ tablespoons lemon juice 2 garlic cloves, minced

Directions:

1. In your blender, combine the red peppers with the parmesan and the rest of the ingredients and pulse well.

2. Divide into cups and serve as a snack.

Nutrition:
calories 200, fat 5.6, fiber 4.5, carbs 12.4, protein 4.6

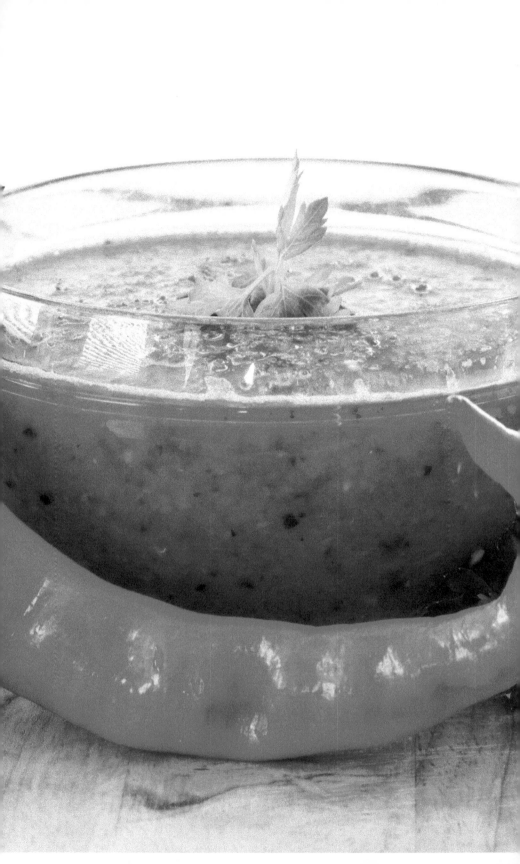

Easy Lemon Chicken Soup

Prep Time: 10 min **Cooking Time:** 10 min **Servings:** 2

Ingredients:

- 1 1/2 lbs chicken breasts, boneless 3 cups chicken stock
- tbsp fresh lemon juice 1/2 tsp garlic powder 1/2 onion, chopped Pepper
- Salt

Directions:

1. Add all ingredients except lemon juice into the inner pot of instant pot and stir well.

2. Seal pot with lid and cook on high for 10 minutes.

3. Once done, allow to release pressure naturally. Remove lid.

4. Remove chicken from pot and shred using a fork. Return shredded chicken to the pot.

5. Stir in lemon juice and serve.

Nutritional Value (Amount per Serving):

Calories 676, Fat 26.2 gCarbohydrates 4.4 gSugar 2.6 gProtein 99.9 g, Cholesterol 303 mg

Leeks Sauté

Prep Time: 10 min   **Cooking Time:** 15 min   **Servings:** 4

Ingredients:

- 2 pounds leeks, sliced
- 2 tablespoons chicken stock
  2 tablespoons tomato paste 1
  tablespoon olive oil
- 2 tablespoons thyme, chopped
  Salt and black pepper to the taste

Directions:

1. Heat up a pan with the oil over medium heat, add the leeks and brown for 5 minutes.

2. Add the rest of the ingredients, toss, increase the heat to medium-high and cook for 10 minutes more.

3. Divide everything between plates and serve as a side dish.

Nutrition:

calories 200, fat 11.4, fiber 5.6, carbs 16.4, protein 3.6

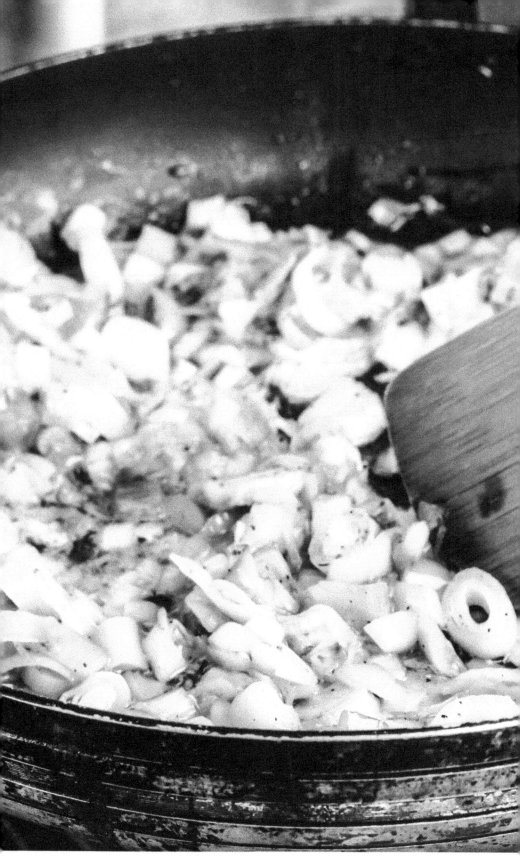

Creamy Chicken Soup

Prep Time: 10 min   **Cooking Time:** 10 min   **Servings:** 6

Ingredients:

- 2 lbs chicken breast, boneless and cut into chunks 8 oz cream cheese
- 2 tbsp taco seasoning 1 cup of salsa
- 2 cups chicken stock
- 28 oz can tomatoes, diced Salt

Directions:

1. Add all ingredients except cream cheese into the instant pot.
2. Seal pot with lid and cook on high pressure 10 for minutes.
3. Once done, allow to release pressure naturally. Remove lid.
4. Remove chicken from pot and shred using a fork. Return shredded chicken to the pot.
5. Add cream cheese and stir well.
6. Serve and enjoy.

Nutritional Value (Amount per Serving):

Calories 471, Fat 24.1 g, Carbohydrates 19.6 g, Sugar 6.2 g, Protein 43.9 g, Cholesterol 157 mg

Chicken Lentil Stew

Prep Time: 10 min   **Cooking Time:** 25 min   **Servings:** 6

Ingredients:

- lbs chicken thighs, boneless & skinless 1 tbsp olive oil
- 1 cup onion, chopped 4 cups chicken stock
- 8 oz green lentils, soak for 1 hour 28 oz can tomato, diced
- Pepper Salt

Directions:

1. Add oil into the inner pot of instant pot and set the pot on sauté mode.
2. Add onion and sauté for 5 minutes.
3. Add the rest of the ingredients and stir well.
4. Seal pot with lid and cook on high for minutes.
5. Once done, release pressure using quick release. Remove lid.
6. Shred chicken using a fork.
7. Stir well and serve.

Nutritional Value (Amount per Serving):

Calories 479, Fat 14.3 g, Carbohydrates 29.8 g, Sugar 5 g, Protein 55.1 g, Cholesterol 135 mg

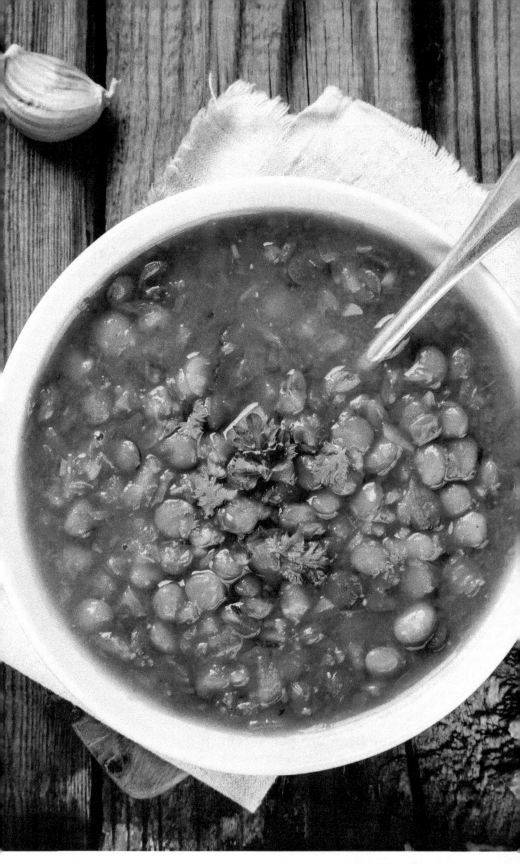

Garlic Squash Broccoli Soup

Prep Time: 10 min   **Cooking Time:** 15 min   **Servings:** 4

Ingredients:

- 1 lb butternut squash, peeled and diced 1 lb broccoli florets
- tsp dried basil 1 tsp paprika
- 1/2 cups vegetable stock 1 tsp garlic, minced
- 1 tbsp olive oil
- 1 onion, chopped Salt

Directions:

1. Add oil into the inner pot of instant pot and set the pot on sauté mode.
2. Add onion and garlic and sauté for 3 minutes.
3. Add remaining ingredients and stir well.
4. Seal pot with lid and cook on high pressure 12 for minutes.
5. Once done, allow to release pressure naturally for 10 minutes then release remaining using quick release. Remove lid.
6. Blend soup using an immersion blender until smooth.
7. Serve and enjoy.

Nutritional Value (Amount per Serving):
Calories 137, Fat 4.1 g, Carbohydrates 24.5 g, Sugar 6.1 g, Protein 5 g, Cholesterol 0 mg

Chicken Rice Soup

Prep Time: 10 min   **Cooking Time:** 9 min   **Servings:** 4

Ingredients:

- 1 lb chicken breast, boneless 2 thyme sprigs
- 1 tsp garlic, chopped 1/4 tsp turmeric
- tbsp olive oil
- tbsp fresh parsley, chopped 2 tbsp fresh lemon juice
- 1/4 cup rice
- 1/2 cup celery, diced 1/2 cup onion, chopped 2 carrots, chopped
- cups vegetable stock Pepper
- Salt

Directions:

1. Add oil into the inner pot of instant pot and set the pot on sauté mode.
2. Add garlic, onion, carrots, and celery and sauté for 3 minutes.
3. Add the rest of the ingredients and stir well.
4. Seal pot with lid and cook on high for 6 minutes.
5. Once done, release pressure using quick release. Remove lid.
6. Shred chicken using a fork.
7. Serve and enjoy.

Nutritional Value (Amount per Serving):

Calories 237, Fat 6.8 g, Carbohydrates 16.6 g, Sugar 3.4 g, Protein 26.2 g, Cholesterol 73 mg

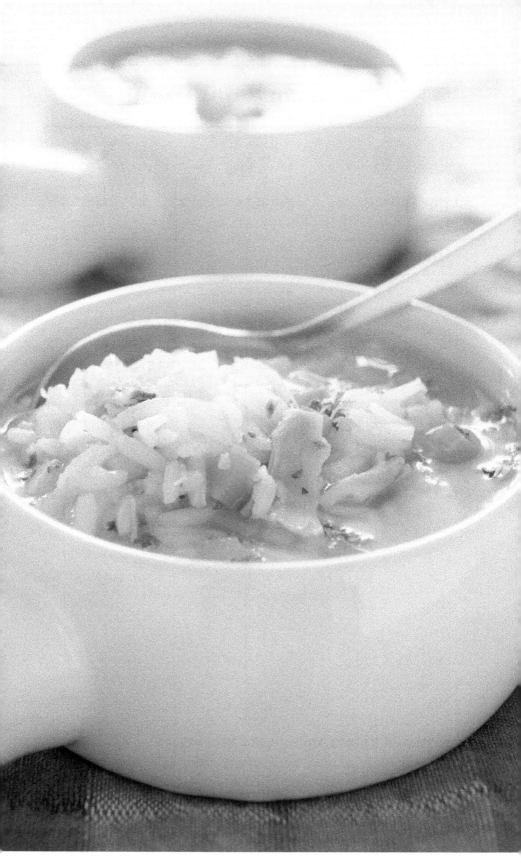

Sausage Potato Soup

Prep Time: 10 min   **Cooking Time:** 20 min   **Servings:** 6

Ingredients:

- 1 lb Italian sausage, crumbled 1 cup half and half
- 1 cup kale, chopped 6 cups chicken stock 1/2 tsp dried oregano
- 3 potatoes, peeled and diced 1 tsp garlic, minced
- 1 onion, chopped 1 tbsp olive oil Pepper
- Salt

Directions:

1. Add oil into the inner pot of instant pot and set the pot on sauté mode.
2. Add sausage, garlic, and onion and sauté for 5 minutes.
3. Add the rest of the ingredients and stir well.
4. Seal pot with lid and cook on high for 15 minutes.
5. Once done, allow to release pressure naturally for 10 minutes then release remaining using quick release. Remove lid.
6. Stir and serve.

Nutritional Value (Amount per Serving):

Calories 426, Fat 29.1 g, Carbohydrates 22.3 g, Sugar 2.8 g, Protein 18.9 g, Cholesterol 78 mg

Easy & Delicious Beef Stew

Prep Time: 10min   **Cooking Time:** 30 min   **Servings:** 4

Ingredients:

*   1 1/2 lbs beef stew meat, cut into cubed 1/2 cup sweet corn
*   1 cup can tomato, crushed 1 cup chicken stock
*   4 carrots, chopped
*   1 onion, chopped 1 tbsp olive oil Pepper
*   Salt

Directions:

1. Add oil into the inner pot of instant pot and set the pot on sauté mode.
2. Add onion and meat and sauté for 5 minutes.
3. Add remaining ingredients and stir well.
4. Seal pot with lid and cook on high pressure 25 for minutes.
5. Once done, allow to release pressure naturally for 10 minutes then release remaining using quick release. Remove lid.
6. Stir and serve.

Nutritional Value (Amount per Serving):

Calories 410, Fat 14.4 g, Carbohydrates 14 g, Sugar 4.8 g, Protein 54.4 g, Cholesterol 152 mg

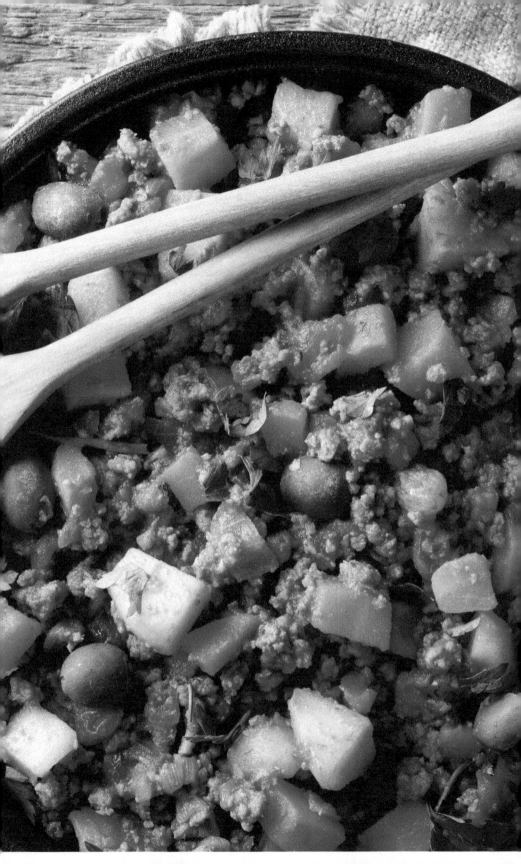

Italian Salsa Chicken Soup

Prep Time: 10 min   **Cooking Time:** 25 min   **Servings:** 6

Ingredients:

- 1 lb chicken breasts, boneless and cut into chunks 3 cups chicken stock
- 8 oz cream cheese 1 1/2 cups salsa
- tsp Italian seasoning
- tbsp fresh parsley, chopped Pepper
- Salt

Directions:

1. Add all ingredients except cream cheese and parsley into the instant pot and stir well.
2. Seal pot with lid and cook on high for 25 minutes.
3. Once done, release pressure using quick release. Remove lid.
4. Remove chicken from pot and shred using a fork. Return shredded chicken to the pot.
5. Add cream cheese and stir well and cook on sauté mode until cheese is melted.
6. Serve and enjoy.

Nutritional Value (Amount per Serving):

Calories 301, Fat 19.4 g, Carbohydrates 5.6 g, Sugar 2.5 g, Protein 26.1 g, Cholesterol 109 mg

Roasted Tomatoes Soup

Prep Time: 10 min   **Cooking Time:** 5 min   **Servings:** 2

Ingredients:

- 14 oz can fire-roasted tomatoes 1 1/2 cups vegetable stock
- 1/4 cup zucchini, grated 1/2 tsp dried oregano 1/2 tsp dried basil
- 1/2 cup heavy cream
- 1/2 cup parmesan cheese, grated 1 cup cheddar cheese, grated Pepper
- Salt

Directions:

1. Add tomatoes, stock, zucchini, oregano, basil, pepper, and salt into the instant pot and stir well.

2. Seal pot with lid and cook on high for 5 minutes.

3. Once done, release pressure using quick release. Remove lid.

4. Set pot on sauté mode. Add heavy cream, parmesan cheese, and cheddar cheese and stir well and cook until cheese is melted.

5. Serve and enjoy.

Nutritional Value (Amount per Serving):

Calories 460, Fat 34.8 g, Carbohydrates 13.5 g, Sugar 6 g, Protein 24.1 g, Cholesterol 117 mg

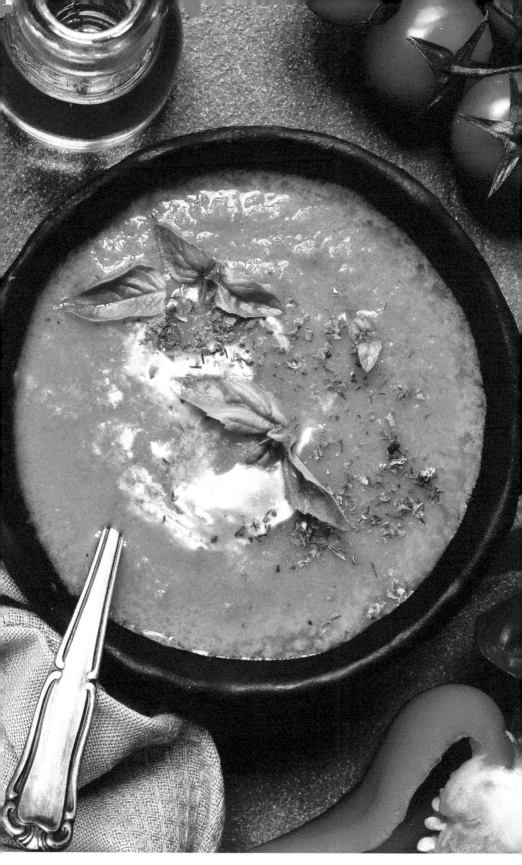

Mussels Soup

Prep Time: 10 min   **Cooking Time:** 3 min   **Servings:** 2

Ingredients:

- oz mussels, cleaned 2 tsp Italian seasoning 2 tbsp olive oil
- 1 cup grape tomatoes, chopped 4 cups chicken stock
- 1/4 cup fish sauce

Directions:

1. Add all ingredients into the inner pot of instant pot and stir well.
2. Seal pot with lid and cook on high for 3 minutes.
3. Once done, release pressure using quick release. Remove lid.
4. Stir well and serve.

Nutritional Value (Amount per Serving):

Calories 256, Fat 18.6 g, Carbohydrates 9.9 g, Sugar 5.5 g, Protein 14.1 g, Cholesterol 27 mg

Mixed Lentil Stew

Prep Time: 10 min   **Cooking Time:** 30 min   **Servings:** 4

Ingredients:

- 1 1/2 cups mixed lentils, rinsed 1/4 cup fresh cilantro, chopped
- 12 oz can chickpeas, drained and rinsed 1 tsp dried oregano
- 1 tsp ground sumac 1 tsp ground ginger 1 tsp garlic powder 1 tbsp ground cumin 1 tbsp paprika
- 28 oz can tomatoes, diced 2 zucchini, chopped
- 1 bell pepper, chopped 3 carrots, chopped
- 1 sweet potato, chopped 1 onion, chopped
- 4 1/2 cups vegetable broth Pepper
- Salt

Directions:

1. Add all ingredients except chickpeas and cilantro into the inner pot of instant pot and stir well.
2. Seal pot with lid and cook on high for minutes.
3. Once done, release pressure using quick release. Remove lid.
4. Add cilantro and chickpeas and stir well.
5. Serve and enjoy.

Nutritional Value (Amount per Serving):

Calories 523, Fat 4.2 g, Carbohydrates 102.6 g, Sugar 16.4 g, Protein 22.5 g, Cholesterol 0 mg

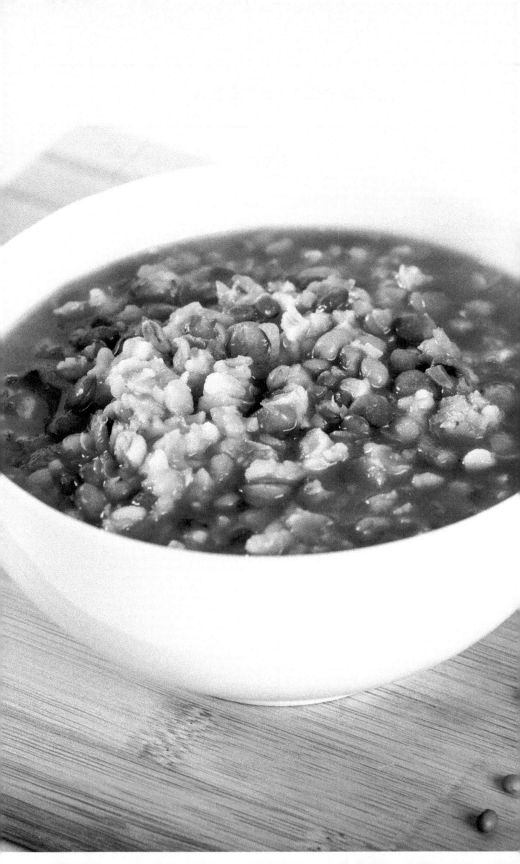

Healthy Cabbage Soup

Prep Time: 10 min   **Cooking Time:** 15 min   **Servings:** 4

Ingredients:

- cabbage head, shredded 4 cups vegetable stock
- 1/4 cup fresh parsley, chopped 1 tbsp garlic, minced
- tbsp olive oil
- 1 onion, chopped 1/2 lb carrots, sliced Pepper
- Salt

Directions:

1. Add oil into the inner pot of instant pot and set the pot on sauté mode.
2. Add onion and garlic and sauté for 5 minutes.
3. Add the rest of the ingredients and stir well.
4. Seal pot with lid and cook on high for 10 minutes.
5. Once done, allow to release pressure naturally for 10 minutes then release remaining using quick release. Remove lid.
6. Stir and serve.

Nutritional Value (Amount per Serving):

Calories 149, Fat 7.4 g, Carbohydrates 20.4 g, Sugar 10.4 g, Protein 3.7 g, Cholesterol 0 mg

Creamy Carrot Tomato Soup

Prep Time: 10 min   **Cooking Time:** 10 min   **Servings:** 6

Ingredients:

- oz can tomatoes, diced 1/2 cup heavy cream
- 1 cup vegetable broth 1 tbsp dried basil
- 1 onion, chopped
- 4 large carrots, peeled and chopped 1/4 cup olive oil
- Pepper Salt

Directions:

1. Add oil into the inner pot of instant pot and set the pot on sauté mode.
2. Add onion and carrots and sauté for 5 minutes.
3. Add the rest of ingredients except heavy cream and stir well.
4. Seal pot with lid and cook on high pressure 5 for minutes.
5. Once done, allow to release pressure naturally. Remove lid.
6. Stir in heavy cream and blend soup using an immersion blender until smooth.
7. Serve and enjoy.

Nutritional Value (Amount per Serving):

Calories 144, Fat 12.4 g, Carbohydrates 7.8 g, Sugar 3.9 g, Protein 1.8 g, Cholesterol 14 mg

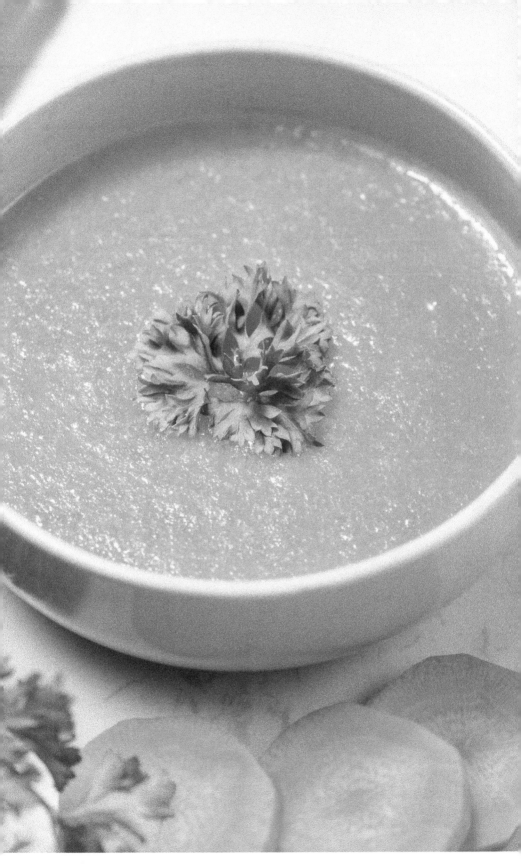

Cheesy Chicken Soup

Prep Time: 10 min   **Cooking Time:** 15 min   **Servings:** 4

Ingredients:

- 12 oz chicken thighs, boneless 1 cup heavy cream
- 2 cups cheddar cheese, shredded 3 cups chicken stock
- 2 tbsp olive oil
- 1/2 cup celery, chopped 1/4 cup hot sauce
- 1 tsp garlic, minced 1/4 cup onion, chopped

Directions:

1. Add all ingredients except cream and cheese into the instant pot and stir well.
2. Seal pot with lid and cook on high pressure 15 for minutes.
3. Once done, allow to release pressure naturally. Remove lid.
4. Shred the chicken using a fork.
5. Add cream and cheese and stir until cheese is melted.
6. Serve and enjoy.

Nutritional Value (Amount per Serving):

Calories 568, Fat 43.6 g, Carbohydrates 3.6 g, Sugar 1.5 g,m Protein 40.1 g, Cholesterol 176 mg

Creamy Cauliflower Soup

Prep Time: 10 min   **Cooking Time:** 23 min   **Servings:** 4

Ingredients:

- 1 lb cauliflower florets, chopped 2 tbsp fresh chives, chopped
- tsp curry powder
- cups vegetable stock 14 oz coconut cream
- 1 onion, chopped
- 1 tbsp garlic, minced 1 tbsp olive oil Pepper
- Salt

Directions:

1. Add oil into the inner pot of instant pot and set the pot on sauté mode.
2. Add onion and garlic and sauté for 3 minutes.
3. Add the rest of the ingredients and stir well.
4. Seal pot with lid and cook on high for 20 minutes.
5. Once done, allow to release pressure naturally for 10 minutes then release remaining using quick release. Remove lid.
6. Blend soup using an immersion blender until smooth.
7. Serve and enjoy.

Nutritional Value (Amount per Serving):

Calories 306, Fat 27.4 g, Carbohydrates 15.6 g, Sugar 7.6 g, Protein 5.3 g, Cholesterol 0 mg

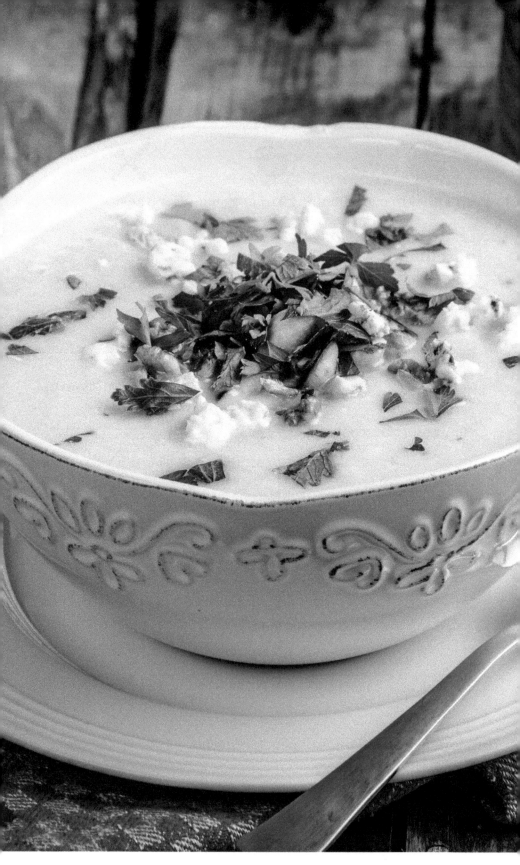

Delicious Okra Chicken Stew

Prep Time: 10 min   **Cooking Time:** 20 min   **Servings:** 4

Ingredients:

- 1 lb chicken breasts, skinless, boneless, and cubed 1 lemon juice
- 1/4 cup fresh parsley, chopped 1 tbsp olive oil
- 12 oz can tomatoes, crushed 1 tsp allspice
- 14 oz okra, chopped 2 cups chicken stock 1 tsp garlic, minced 1 onion, chopped Pepper
- Salt

Directions:

1. Add oil into the inner pot of instant pot and set the pot on sauté mode.
2. Add chicken and onion and sauté until chicken is lightly brown about 5 minutes.
3. Add remaining ingredients except for the parsley and stir well.
4. Seal pot with lid and cook on high pressure 15 for minutes.
5. Once done, allow to release pressure naturally for 10 minutes then release remaining using quick release. Remove lid.
6. Stir well and serve.

Nutritional Value (Amount per Serving):

Calories 326, Fat 12.6 g, Carbohydrates 15.8 g, Sugar 6.2 g, Protein 36.4 g, Cholesterol 101 mg

Healthy Vegetable Soup

Prep Time: 10 min   **Cooking Time:** 15 min   **Servings:** 4

Ingredients:

- 1 cup can tomatoes, chopped 1 small zucchini, diced
- 3 oz kale, sliced
- 1 tbsp garlic, chopped
- 5 button mushrooms, sliced 2 carrots, peeled and sliced
- 2 celery sticks, sliced 1/2 red chili, sliced
- 1 onion, diced 1 tbsp olive oil 1 bay leaf
- 4 cups vegetable stock 1/4 tsp salt

Directions:

1. Add oil into the inner pot of instant pot and set the pot on sauté mode.
2. Add carrots, celery, onion, and salt and cook for 2-3 minutes.
3. Add mushrooms and chili and cook for 2 minutes.
4. Add remaining ingredients and stir everything well.
5. Seal pot with lid and cook on high for 10 minutes.
6. Once done, allow to release pressure naturally for 10 minutes then release remaining using quick release. Remove lid.
7. Stir well and serve.

Nutritional Value (Amount per Serving):

Calories 100, Fat 3.8 g, Carbohydrates 15.1 g, Sugar 6.6 g, Protein 3.5 g, Cholesterol 0 mg

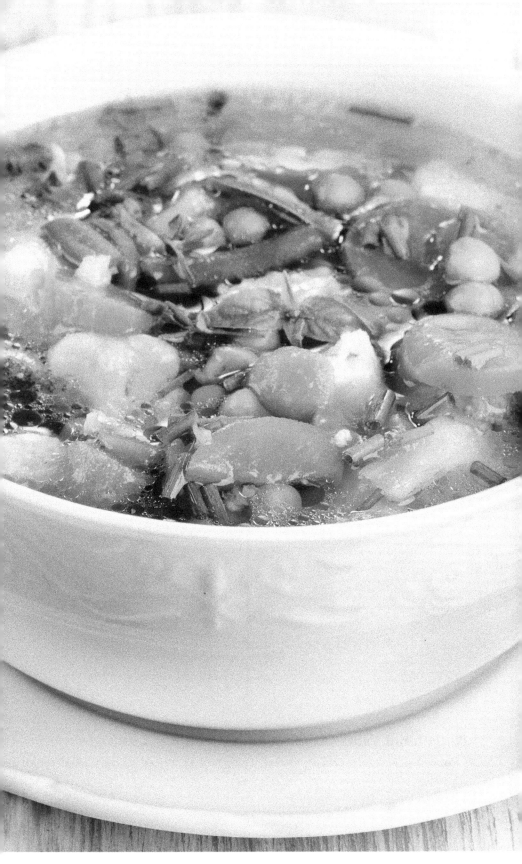

Spinach Chicken Stew

Prep Time: 10 min   **Cooking Time:**25 min   **Servings:** 4

Ingredients:

- 2 cups spinach, chopped
- 1 lb chicken breasts, skinless, boneless, and cut into chunks 1/2 cup can tomato, crushed
- 1 cup chicken stock 1 onion, chopped
- 1 tbsp olive oil Pepper
- Salt

Directions:

1. Add oil into the inner pot of instant pot and set the pot on sauté mode.
2. Add chicken and onion and sauté for 5 minutes.
3. Add remaining ingredients and stir well.
4. Seal pot with lid and cook on low for 20 minutes.
5. Once done, allow to release pressure naturally for 10 minutes then release remaining using quick release. Remove lid.
6. Stir well and serve.

Nutritional Value (Amount per Serving):

Calories 266, Fat 12.2 g, Carbohydrates 4.2 g, Sugar 1.4 g, Protein 33.9 g, Cholesterol 101 mg

Spinach Lentil Soup

Prep Time: 10 min   **Cooking Time:** 30 min   **Servings:** 4

Ingredients:

- 4 cups spinach
- 2 cups green lentils
- 4 cups vegetable stock 1 tsp Italian seasoning
- 14 oz can tomatoes, chopped 2 tsp thyme, chopped
- 1 tsp garlic, minced 1 carrot, chopped
- onion, chopped
- celery stalks, chopped Pepper
- Salt

Directions:

1. Add all ingredients except spinach into the inner pot of instant pot and stir well.
2. Seal pot with lid and cook on high for 25 minutes.
3. Once done, allow to release pressure naturally for 10 minutes then release remaining using quick release. Remove lid.
4. Add spinach and stir well and cook on sauté mode for 5 minutes.
5. Stir well and serve.

Nutritional Value (Amount per Serving):

Calories 398, Fat 1.7 g, Carbohydrates 69.8 g, Sugar 8.3 g, Protein 27.5 g, Cholesterol 1 mg

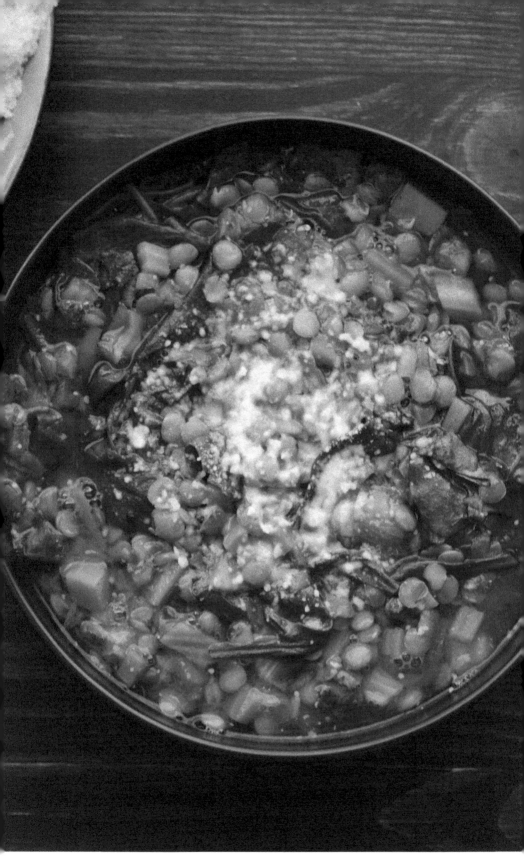

Basil Broccoli Soup

Prep Time: 10 min **Cooking Time:** 15 min **Servings:** 6

Ingredients:

- 1 lb broccoli florets 1 tbsp olive oil
- 1 tsp chili powder 1 tsp dried basil
- 6 cups vegetable stock 1 onion, chopped
- 2 leeks, chopped Pepper
- Salt

Directions:

1. Add oil into the inner pot of instant pot and set the pot on sauté mode.
2. Add onion and leek and sauté for 5 minutes.
3. Add the rest of the ingredients and stir well.
4. Seal pot with lid and cook on high for 10 minutes.
5. Once done, allow to release pressure naturally for 10 minutes then release remaining using quick release. Remove lid.
6. Blend soup using an immersion blender until smooth.
7. Serve and enjoy.

Nutritional Value (Amount per Serving):

Calories 79, Fat 2.9 g, Carbohydrates 12.1 g, Sugar 4 g, Protein 3.2 g, Cholesterol 0 mg

Basil Zucchini Soup

Prep Time: 10 min   **Cooking Time:** 15 min   **Servings:** 4

Ingredients:

- zucchini, chopped
- 2 tbsp fresh basil, chopped
- 30 oz vegetable stock 1 tbsp garlic, minced
- 2 cups tomatoes, chopped 1 1/2 cup corn
- 1 onion, chopped
- 1 celery stalk, chopped 1 tbsp olive oil
- Pepper Salt

Directions:

1. Add oil into the inner pot of instant pot and set the pot on sauté mode.
2. Add onion and garlic and sauté for 5 minutes.
3. Add remaining ingredients except for basil and stir well.
4. Seal pot with lid and cook on high for 10 minutes.
5. Once done, allow to release pressure naturally for 10 minutes then release remaining using quick release. Remove lid.
6. Stir in basil and serve.

Nutritional Value (Amount per Serving):

Calories 139, Fat 4.8 g, Carbohydrates 23 g, Sugar 8.7 g, Protein 5.2 g, Cholesterol 0 mg

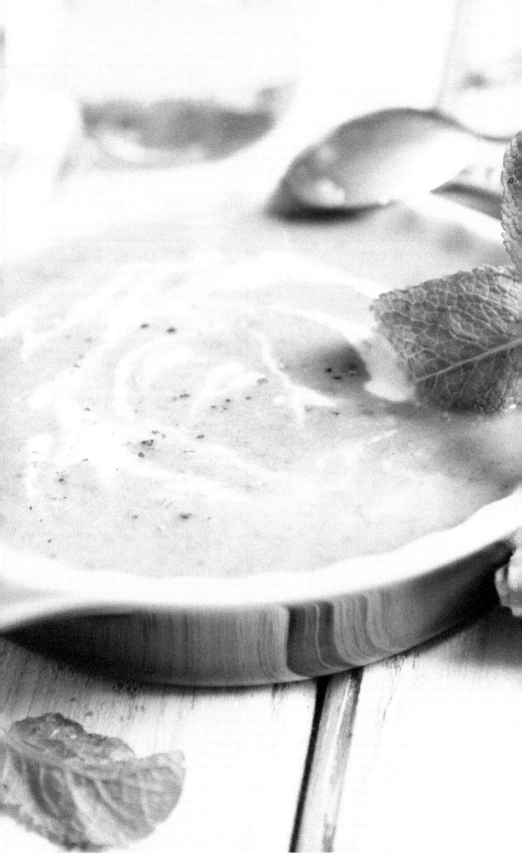

Mushroom Carrot Soup

Prep Time: 10 min   **Cooking Time:** 20 min   **Servings:** 4

Ingredients:

- 16 oz mushrooms, sliced 1 carrot, chopped
- 4 cups vegetable stock 1 tsp dried thyme
- 1 tbsp garlic, minced
- 1 onion, chopped
- 1 celery stalk, chopped 1 tbsp olive oil
- Pepper Salt

Directions:

1. Add oil into the inner pot of instant pot and set the pot on sauté mode.
2. Add onion, garlic, celery, and carrot and sauté for 5 minutes.
3. Add mushrooms and sauté for 5 minutes.
4. Add the rest of the ingredients and stir well.
5. Seal pot with lid and cook on high for 10 minutes.
6. Once done, allow to release pressure naturally for 10 minutes then release remaining using quick release. Remove lid.
7. Blend soup using an immersion blender until smooth.
8. Serve and enjoy.

Nutritional Value (Amount per Serving):

Calories 82, Fat 4 g, Carbohydrates 9.7 g, Sugar 4.6 g,m, Protein 4.6 g, Cholesterol 0 mg

Tomato Pepper Soup

Prep Time: 10 min   **Cooking Time:** 20 min   **Servings:** 4

Ingredients:

- lb tomatoes, chopped
- red bell peppers, chopped 1/2 tsp red pepper flakes 1/2 tbsp dried basil
- 1 tsp garlic powder
- 6 cups vegetable stock 2 celery stalk, chopped 3 tbsp tomato paste
- 1 onion, chopped 2 tbsp olive oil Pepper
- Salt

Directions:

1. Add oil into the inner pot of instant pot and set the pot on sauté mode.
2. Add onion, red pepper flakes, basil, and garlic powder and sauté for 5 minutes.
3. Add remaining ingredients and stir well.
4. Seal pot with lid and cook on high for 15 minutes.
5. Once done, allow to release pressure naturally for 10 minutes then release remaining using quick release. Remove lid.
6. Blend soup using an immersion blender until smooth.
7. Serve and enjoy.

Nutritional Value (Amount per Serving):

Calories 134, Fat 7.7 g, Carbohydrates 16 g, Sugar 10 g, Protein 3.2 g, Cholesterol 0 mg

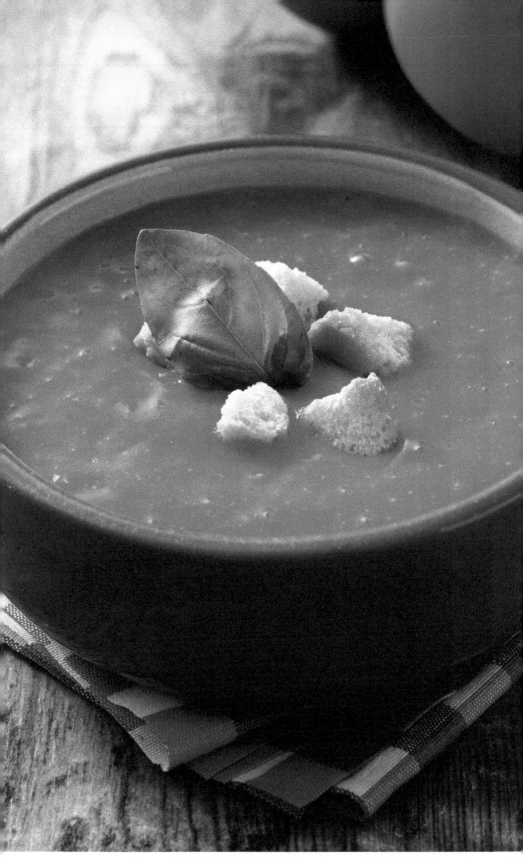

Tomato Chickpeas Stew

Prep Time: 10 min   **Cooking Time:** 25 min   **Servings:** 4

Ingredients:

- 1 lb can chickpeas, rinsed and drained 18 oz can tomatoes, chopped
- 1/2 tsp red pepper flakes 2 tbsp olive oil
- tsp dried oregano 1 tsp garlic, minced 1 onion, chopped Pepper
- Salt

Directions:

1. Add oil into the inner pot of instant pot and set the pot on sauté mode.
2. Add onion and garlic and sauté for 5 minutes.
3. Add remaining ingredients and stir well.
4. Seal pot with lid and cook on high pressure 20 for minutes.
5. Once done, allow to release pressure naturally for 10 minutes then release remaining using quick release. Remove lid.
6. Serve and enjoy.

Nutritional Value (Amount per Serving):

Calories 236 Fat 8.4 g, Carbohydrates 35.3 g, Sugar 5.6 g, Protein 7.2 g, Cholesterol 0 mg

Italian Chicken Stew

Prep Time: 10 min   **Cooking Time:** 12 min   **Servings:** 6

Ingredients:

- lb chicken breasts, boneless 2 potatoes, peeled and diced 3 carrots, cut into chunks
- celery stalks, cut into chunks 1 onion, diced
- 1 tsp garlic, minced 1 tsp ground sage 1/2 tsp thyme
- 1/2 tsp dried basil
- cups chicken stock Pepper
- Salt

Directions:

1. Add all ingredients into the inner pot of instant pot and stir well.
2. Seal pot with lid and cook on high for 12 minutes.
3. Once done, allow to release pressure naturally for 10 minutes then release remaining using quick release. Remove lid.
4. Remove chicken from pot and shred using a fork. Return shredded chicken to the pot.
5. Stir well and serve.

Nutritional Value (Amount per Serving):

Calories 220, Fat 6 g, Carbohydrates 16.7 g, Sugar 3.5 g, Protein 23.9 g, Cholesterol 67 mg

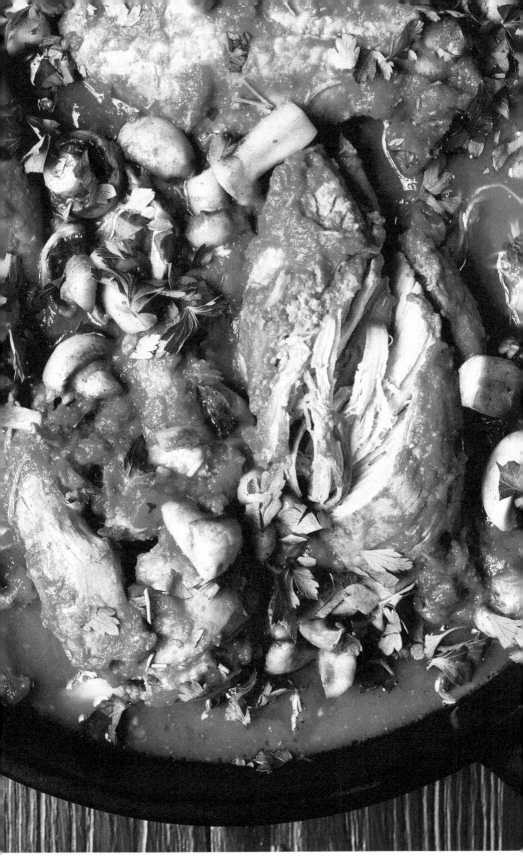

Healthy Lentil Soup

Prep Time: 10 min   **Cooking Time:** 30 min   **Servings:** 8

Ingredients:

- 1 cup red lentils
- 1 tsp fresh lemon juice 8 cups vegetable broth 1 tsp ground cumin
- 1 tbsp garlic, chopped 2 carrots, chopped
- 1 onion, chopped
- 1 split pea Pepper Salt

Directions:

1. Add all ingredients except lemon juice into the instant pot and stir well.
2. Seal pot with lid and cook on high pressure 30 for minutes.
3. Once done, allow to release pressure naturally. Remove lid.
4. Stir in Lemont juice and serve.

Nutritional Value (Amount per Serving):

Calories 121, Fat 0.4 g, Carbohydrates 21.8 g, Sugar 4 g, Protein 7.1 g, Cholesterol 0 mg

Chicken Noodle Soup

Prep Time: 10 min   **Cooking Time:** 10 min   **Servings:** 6

Ingredients:

- 6 cups cooked chicken, shredded 1 tbsp garlic, minced
- 8 oz whole wheat noodles 1 bell pepper, chopped
- 1 carrot, peeled and sliced
- 6 cups chicken stock 2 celery stalks, sliced 1 onion, chopped
- 3 tbsp rice vinegar
- 2 1/2 cups cabbage, shredded 2 tbsp fresh ginger, grated
- 2 tbsp soy sauce

Directions:

1. Add all ingredients into the inner pot of instant pot and stir well.
2. Seal pot with lid and cook on high for 10 minutes.
3. Once done, release pressure using quick release. Remove lid.
4. Stir well and serve.

Nutritional Value (Amount per Serving):

Calories 389, Fat 6.4 g, Carbohydrates 22.9 g, Sugar 4.2 g, Protein 49.3 g, Cholesterol 128 mg

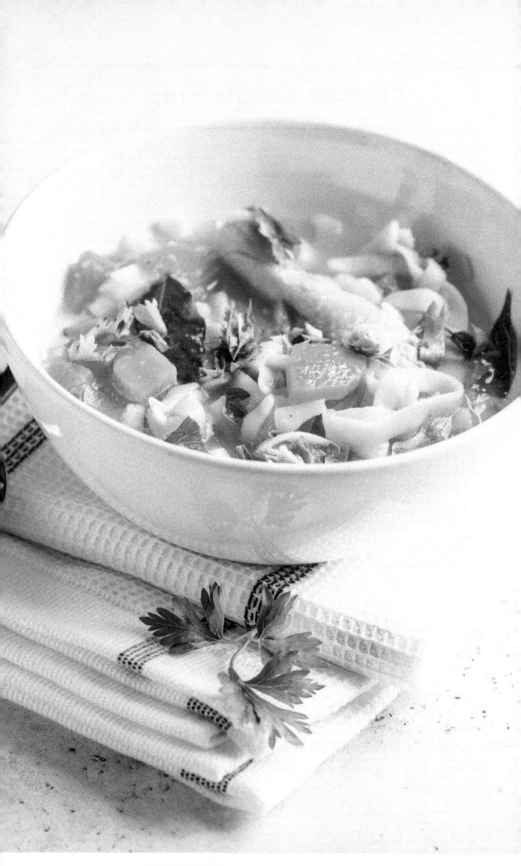

Spinach Cauliflower Soup

Prep Time: 10 min **Cooking Time:** 10 min **Servings:** 2

Ingredients:

- 1 cup cauliflower, chopped 3 cups spinach, chopped
- 1 tsp garlic powder 2 tbsp olive oil
- 3 cups vegetable broth 1/2 cup heavy cream Pepper
- Salt

Directions:

1. Add all ingredients except cream into the inner pot of instant pot and stir well.
2. Seal pot with lid and cook on high for 10 minutes.
3. Once done, release pressure using quick release. Remove lid.
4. Stir in cream and blend soup using an immersion blender until smooth.
5. Serve and enjoy.

Nutritional Value (Amount per Serving):

Calories 309, Fat 27.4 g, Carbohydrates 7.5 g, Sugar 2.8 g, Protein 10.4 g, Cholesterol 41 mg

Nutritious Kidney Bean Soup

Prep Time: 10 min   **Cooking Time:** 1h 40m   **Servings:** 8

Ingredients:

- cups red kidney beans, soaked overnight & drain 1/4 cup fresh parsley, chopped
- 6 cups of water 1/4 cup olive oil
- 1 1/2 tbsp tomato paste 2 bell peppers, chopped 2 carrots, chopped
- 1 tbsp garlic, minced 1 onion, chopped
- 1 tsp salt

Directions:

1. Add oil into the inner pot of instant pot and set the pot on sauté mode.
2. Add garlic and onion and sauté until onion is softened.
3. Add carrots and bell peppers and sauté for 3-5 minutes.
4. Add beans, parsley, tomato paste, water, and salt and stir everything well.
5. Seal pot with lid and cook on high for 1 hour 40 minutes.
6. Once done, release pressure using quick release. Remove lid.
7. Stir well and serve.

Nutritional Value (Amount per Serving):

Calories 312, Fat 7.2 g, Carbohydrates 48.4 g, Sugar 4.7 g, Protein 16.4 g, Cholesterol 0 mg

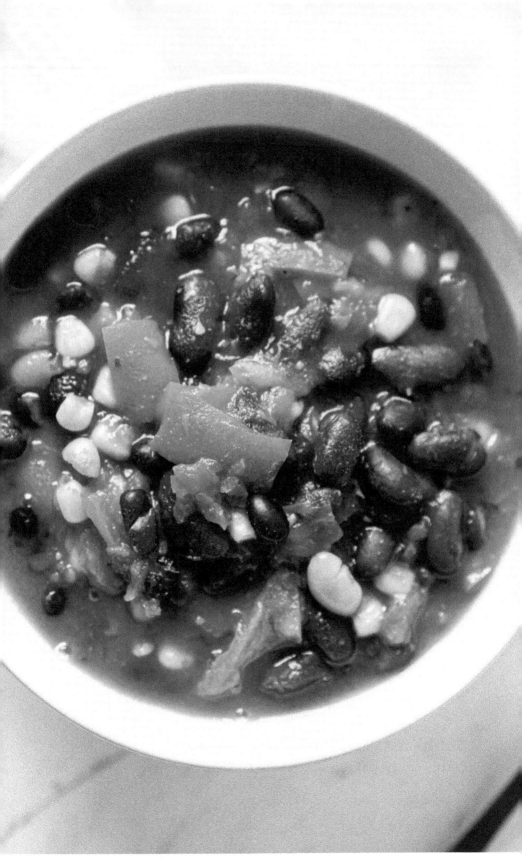

Hearty Pork Stew

Prep Time: 10 min   **Cooking Time:** 15 min   **Servings:** 4

Ingredients:

- 1/2 lb ground pork
- 1 tbsp fresh lemon juice
- 1/4 cup fresh parsley, chopped 1 cup of water
- 14 oz can tomatoes, chopped
- 2 cups can navy beans, rinsed and drained 3 medium potatoes, peeled and diced
- 1 tbsp garlic, chopped 1/2 tsp red pepper flakes 1 tsp dried thyme
- 1 carrot, peeled and diced 2 celery sticks, diced
- 1 onion, diced 2 tbsp olive oil 2 tsp salt

Directions:

1. Add oil into the inner pot of instant pot and set the pot on sauté mode.
2. Add carrot, celery, onion, and 1 tsp salt and sauté for 5 minutes.
3. Add meat and cook for 2-4 minutes.
4. Add remaining ingredients except for lemon juice and parsley and stir everything well.
5. Seal pot with lid and cook on high for 6 minutes.
6. Once done, allow to release pressure naturally for 10 minutes then release remaining using quick release. Remove lid.
7. Add lemon juice and stir well.
8. Garnish with parsley and serve.

Nutritional Value (Amount per Serving):

Calories 446, Fat 9.9 g, Carbohydrates 62.6 g, Sugar 7.8 g, Protein 29.1 g, Cholesterol 41 mg

Chili Chicken Soup

Prep Time: 10 min   **Cooking Time:** 10 min   **Servings:** 2

Ingredients:

- 1/2 lb cook chicken, shredded 7 oz can tomatoes, chopped 1/4 tsp cayenne
- 1/4 tsp chili powder
- 1/2 cup mozzarella cheese, shredded 2 tbsp hot sauce
- 1 tbsp olive oil
- 1 1/2 cups chicken stock Pepper
- Salt

Directions:

1. Add all ingredients into the inner pot of instant pot and stir well.
2. Seal pot with lid and cook on high for 10 minutes.
3. Once done, allow to release pressure naturally. Remove lid.
4. Stir well and serve.

Nutritional Value (Amount per Serving):

Calories 294, Fat 13.9 g, Carbohydrates 26.7 g, Sugar 24.4 g, Protein 17.7 g, Cholesterol 75 mg

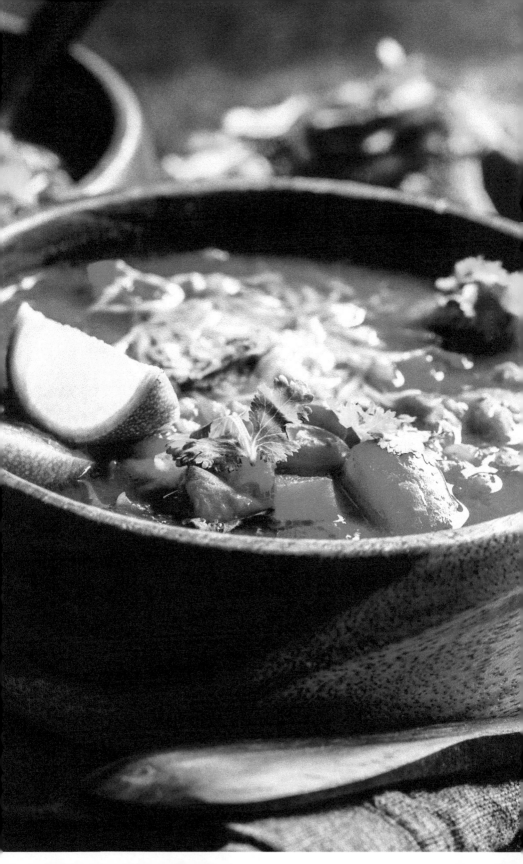

Kidney Bean Soup

Prep Time: 10 min   **Cooking Time:** 15 min   **Servings:** 6

Ingredients:

- 1 lb kidney beans, soaked overnight and drained 1 tsp paprika
- 7 cups chicken stock 1 tomato, chopped
- 1 tbsp garlic, chopped 1 onion, chopped
- tbsp olive oil Pepper
- Salt

Directions:

1. Add oil into the inner pot of instant pot and set the pot on sauté mode.
2. Add garlic and onion and sauté for 3 minutes.
3. Add remaining ingredients and stir well.
4. Seal pot with lid and cook on high for 12 minutes.
5. Once done, allow to release pressure naturally for 10 minutes then release remaining using quick release. Remove lid.
6. Stir and serve.

Nutritional Value (Amount per Serving):

Calories 299, Fat 3.9 g, Carbohydrates 50 g, Sugar 3.5 g, Protein 18.3 g, Cholesterol 0 mg

Pepper Pumpkin Soup

Prep Time: 10 min   **Cooking Time:** 6 min   **Servings:** 6

Ingredients:

- 2 cups pumpkin puree 1 onion, chopped
- 4 cups vegetable broth 1/4 tsp nutmeg
- 1/4 cup red bell pepper, chopped 1/8 tsp thyme, dried
- 1/2 tsp salt

Directions:

1. Add all ingredients into the instant pot and stir well.
2. Seal pot with lid and cook on high for 6 minutes.
3. Once done, allow to release pressure naturally for 5 minutes then release remaining using quick release. Remove lid.
4. Blend soup using an immersion blender until smooth.
5. Serve and enjoy.

Nutritional Value (Amount per Serving):

Calories 63, Fat 1.2 g, Carbohydrates 9.4 g, Sugar 4.2 g, Protein 4.4 g, Cholesterol 0 mg

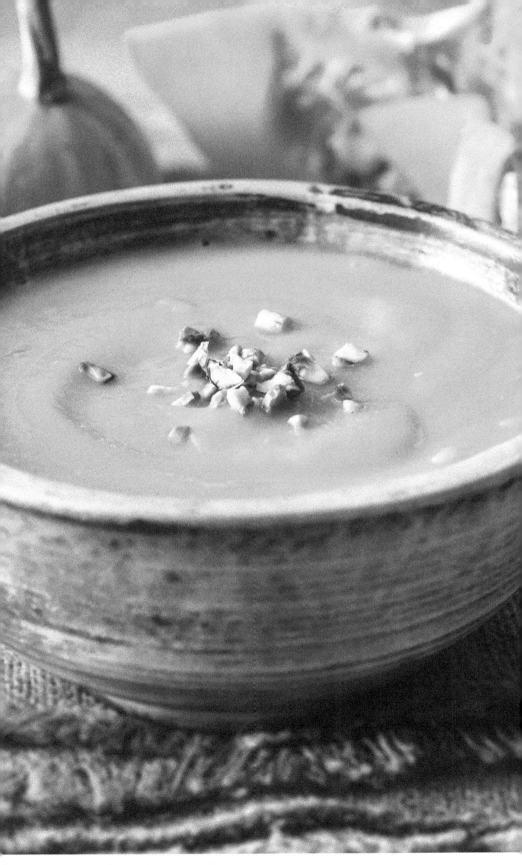

CONCLUSION

Thank you for reaching the end of this book, "Mediterranean Diet Cookbook for Beginners". I hope you enjoyed reading it as much as I had while writing it. As you can now see, the Mediterranean diet is not a restrictive one and it's so easy to follow. As you can also see, it's all about living a healthy and happy life – it's not about being skinny or losing weight – it's about how to adjust your diet to make you healthier and happier.

In comparison to other diets out there, Mediterranean Diet is low in saturated fat, cholesterol, trans-fat and sodium. It also lows in total fat, polyunsaturated fat, and has a moderate amount of carbohydrates. So even though Mediterranean Diet is low in total fat, it has a moderate amount of saturated fat and a nice amount of monounsaturated fats. It is extremely high in dietary fiber, which means you get all the fiber you need with this diet.

The Mediterranean diet actually is more positively defined by dietary patterns than by single food items. The diet emphasizes eating primarily plant-derived foods with olive oil. However, this diet doesn't prescribe that you must eat a particular food.

The Mediterranean diet emphasizes getting more vegetables, fruits, grains, beans, seeds, nuts, legumes, herbs, and spices. It also stresses eating fish and seafood (no red meat usually) and poultry, as well as using wine in moderation. It is all about balance and moderation, and it's about eating fresh, unprocessed foods, plenty of fruits and vegetables, whole grains, beans, seeds, nuts, legumes, herbs and spices. It is about being active every day and not eating too much. The Mediterranean diet avoids processed foods preferring to use fresh foods. You can eat so many wonderful and delicious dishes from the Mediterranean diet, and now you can have all the recipes you need in "Mediterranean Diet Cookbook for Beginners" to help change your lifestyle for the better.

Here are some tips for you to continually maintain this diet:

1. Balance your diet
2. Eat more frequently, but in smaller portions
3. Don't skip meals
4. Maintain a healthy consistency in your meals
5. Give it time to adjust your body to the new foods and ingredients
6. Make the change realistic and achievable
7. Eliminate processed and refined foods from your diet
8. Don't be afraid of eating a variety of foods
9. Don't deprive yourself of treats
10. Keep a food diary
11. Don't be too hard on yourself
12. Take a walk after meals
13. Go for a swim or do some more exercise
14. Stay positive. You're worth this diet and the new lifestyle it has to offer you.

I would like you to think about what you can do with the knowledge that you now have. The main thing is to go out and try the recipes. Cook them for your loved ones, or for friends and family. Cook and enjoy. You have no obligation to follow what I have written here.

The other best thing to do is try to cook Mediterranean dishes yourself – thinking about your diet changes and see how delicious the food can be.

The Mediterranean diet will change the way you look in a matter of days. It will improve your bowel movements and digestion in a matter of days. It will keep you fuller for longer. It will increase your energy and improve your mood. These things happen to everyone who tries this diet, if you follow it correctly. Thank you for reading my book, and I hope that it will help you change your life and that of your loved ones in a very positive way.

To your health and happiness.

Again, thank you for your time. So now you have a great way to start your healthy Mediterranean lifestyle.